FOREWORD

Today's practice of forensic science demands close attention to detail, analytical skill, and perseverance. Scientists work in laboratories with case backlogs under time pressure, often with limited resources. Every year the need for more forensic analysis increases, all within a climate of media scrutiny and a standard of perfectionism.

The Crime Scene: How Forensic Science Works provides a complete overview of the criminal investigative process. Starting at the crime scene, the authors review how evidence is collected, culminating in its presentation in the courtroom. Each chapter provides a foundation in a forensic discipline. The cumulative effect is that of an introductory education in the forensic sciences.

Readers will appreciate the clear examples provided throughout. For students in search of career information, the book provides a realistic job preview. For criminal justice professionals, including attorneys, prosecutors, and judges, the book will serve as a useful resource. For law enforcement professionals, the book reveals the basics of procedures used in the lab. For those in specific academic programs, the book serves as a supplemental text. For all readers, *The Crime Scene: How Forensic Science Works* is a great find!

Importantly, Dale and Becker provide insight into the big picture of the total forensic process. The book fills a critical void in this regard. The forensic sciences are composed of many specific academic disciplines and few have attempted an overview of the continuous process. Using insight derived from their collaborative research, Dale and Becker champion a team-based approach.

A fictional case is highlighted throughout the book that demonstrates the twists and turns of the investigative process from first responder to autopsy and from lab work to conviction. The reader follows workers in their roles, experiencing the everyday insights and frustrations. In addition, experts in autopsy, forensic legal issues, and educational programs have contributed to the technical chapters in the book. Photographs provide stunning visuals to supplement the text.

There is no room for human error in the forensic sciences; and no resource would be complete without reference to the role of quality assurance. There is an emphasis on quality on every page. The Crime Scene Process Flow Chart (centerpiece) shows how each step along the way undergoes a quality review. A detailed appendix contains the international guidelines and quality standards needed for laboratory accreditation. Other treasures can be found as well, including recommended academic programs, Web and print resources, complete technical documents describing the dynamics within forensic laboratories, and a detailed description of the job of forensic scientist.

I heartily recommend *The Crime Scene: How Forensic Science Works.*

—Carl M. Selavka, Ph.D., D-ABC
Former Director, Massachusetts State Police Crime Laboratory System

W. Mark Dale, M.B.A., and Wendy S. Becker, Ph.D.
Northeast Regional Forensics Institute

THE CRIME SCENE:
HOW FORENSIC SCIENCE WORKS

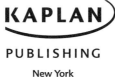

KAPLAN

PUBLISHING

New York

This publication is designed to provide accurate and authoritative information in regard to the subject matter covered. It is sold with the understanding that the publisher is not engaged in rendering legal, accounting, or other professional service. If legal advice or other expert assistance is required, the services of a competent professional should be sought.

Vice President and Publisher: Maureen McMahon
Editorial Director: Jennifer Farthing
Acquisitions Editor: Allyson Rogers Bozeth
Development Editor: Allyson Rogers Bozeth
Contributing Editor: Carolyn Hanson
Production Editor: Fred Urfer
Production Designer: Ivelisse Robles
Typesetter: Todd Bowman
Cover Designer: Rod Hernandez

Published by Kaplan Publishing, a division of Kaplan, Inc.
1 Liberty Plaza, 24th Floor
New York, NY 10006

Printed in the United States of America

December 2007
10 9 8 7 6 5 4 3 2 1

ISBN-13: 978-1-4277-9632-5

Kaplan Publishing books are available at special quantity discounts to use for sales promotions, employee premiums, or educational purposes. Please email our Special Sales Department to order or for more information at *kaplanpublishing@kaplan.com,* or write to Kaplan Publishing, 1 Liberty Plaza, 24th Floor, New York, NY 10006.

TABLE OF CONTENTS

Acknowledgments

We are deeply grateful to our colleagues for their assistance throughout the publication process. We thank the contributing authors for their research and a job well done. Jackie Higgins Chan and Diane Scala-Barnett, M.D., contributed to "Evidence from the Autopsy." Jackie is a DNA scientist with the FBI; previously, she was an autopsy assistant with the city of Toledo, Ohio. Diane Scala-Barnett, M.D., provided additional technical review; she is deputy coroner, Lucas County, Toledo, Ohio. Robert Conflitti provided information for "Legal Issues." Previously, he was a prosecutor for Orange County, New York. Donald Orokos is associate director of the Forensic Molecular Biology Program, operations manager for Northeast Regional Forensic Institute (NERFI), and instructor in biology at the University at Albany. Don provided information for "Becoming a Forensic Professional." Jamie Belrose was a DNA scientist with the New York City Office of the Chief Medical Examiner DNA Laboratory; currently, she is an instructor for the Northeast Regional Forensic Institute DNA Academy program at the University at Albany. Jamie helped obtain the extensive photographs that supplement the book.

Our editorial team at Kaplan helped to bring the project to fruition. Most notably, Jennifer Farthing, editorial director, provided expert guidance throughout the publication process. Allyson Rogers Bozeth, acquisitions editor, was our very first contact at Kaplan. Contributing editor Carolyn Hanson used her mind-reading ability to anticipate what we really wanted to say, and helped us say it better. Andy Jacknick provided editorial assistance and Fred Urfer was production editor.

Writing this book has been a joy. We thank our families for their encouragement throughout, especially Kathy, Mike, Amy, Molly (Mark), Matt, Dave, Betsy, Nancy, and Clara Jane (Wendy) for their ever-present love and support.

INTRODUCTION

"The Crime Scene: How Forensic Science Works *provides a solid introduction to the forensic sciences and crime scene work that can be understood by the nonforensic scientist, the lawyer, and the layperson.*"

—Max Houck

Director, Forensic Science Initiative, Research Office Manager, Forensic Research and Business Development, College of Business and Economics, West Virginia University

A terrible crime has been committed. The evening news provides sketchy detail. Behind the scenes, police rush evidence to the forensic science lab. There, scientists carefully analyze tiny fibers, blood, and other trace evidence using sophisticated equipment and testing methods. Their meticulous work is ultimately used in court to convict the guilty.

The Crime Scene: How Forensic Science Works provides an overview of events that take place from the crime scene to the courtroom. Media and the entertainment industry have sparked public interest in forensic science through dramatic television shows and documentaries, but all the material collected at the crime scene cannot be scientifically examined and cases are not solved in 60 minutes. Simply put, the forensic science shown on prime time is not reality.

Solving crimes is important and satisfying work involving teams of dedicated professionals. In truth, police agencies are limited in resource capacity. Only one-third of DNA cases submitted to forensic laboratories in the United States are currently analyzed, while the number of cases submitted grows each year. Expert data systems, robotics, and batch processing increase lab productivity and quality, but also increase the need for extensive employee training. Most forensic scientists work within the quasi-military structure of police organizations. Local, state, and federal budgets for investigating forensic crimes must compete with more visible crime-fighting resources, such as patrol officers and vehicles.

A realistic job preview is a technique used to highlight the good, the bad, and the ugly about a job. Realistic job previews help to both increase future organizational commitment and decrease job turnover. Clear, specific, and complete information reduces the false expectations that prospective employees have about the nature of a job.

The Crime Scene: How Forensic Science Works provides a realistic preview of the job of forensic scientist, by walking through the steps that ultimately help solve thousands of criminal cases every day. Forensic science is an exciting and rewarding career. One essential piece of probative evidence developed in the laboratory can solve a case by identifying or excluding a suspect. Yet there are many small, mundane, yet important tasks that are also part of the job.

Forensic scientists must work under tremendous pressure without committing any errors and this is a heavy burden to bear. Scientific casework is reviewed many times before being reported to detectives and the criminal justice community. There are serious consequences if a mistake is made. Guilty parties may continue to commit violent crimes or the wrong person may be convicted. The entire community pays the price for one error made by a forensic scientist.

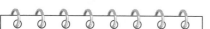

It is important to know one true fact: Forensic scientists are scientists first. Only after becoming a scientist can one pursue a career as a forensic scientist.

This demand for both productivity and error-free work necessitates a highly selective recruitment process. Only the best make the team. A solid foundation in biology, chemistry, and math is required to enter most forensic disciplines. Scientists are screened through extensive background checks, similar to law enforcement. Past behavior that includes criminal offenses, drug use or alcohol abuse, chronic financial difficulty, or gaps in employment will eliminate candidates from consideration.

Historically, forensic science remained hidden in the background of criminal investigations, supporting the conclusions of detectives but seldom providing the "smoking gun." One of the most definitive types of evidence in police work was a physical match—a fractured piece of glass from an automotive headlight lens or a fingerprint that placed the suspect at the scene of the crime. Experienced forensic scientists would proudly say, "This case was solved with a physical match." Today, the DNA technology used in the Combined DNA Index System (CODIS) and computerized imaging databases, such as Automated Fingerprint Identification System (AFIS) and National Integrated Ballistic Information Network (NIBIN), have expanded the scope and efficiency of forensic science. This dramatic revolution has just begun. Fewer than 50 cells of human biological material

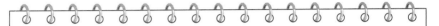

MARK'S STORY

Largely through serendipity and timing, I entered the field of forensic science. I was a patrol sergeant in Long Island, New York, in a very busy police station that investigated a wide variety of criminal activity that generated a vast array of evidence. But I also had a degree in biology and often wondered what actually took place in the crime lab. One day I received a call from the personnel officer at New York State Police headquarters. "Sergeant Dale, we did a computer search of all employees and notice you have a degree in biology. We would like to transfer you to our forensic laboratory. By the way, we want you to start next week! Will you accept this transfer?" Without a moment's hesitation, I jumped at the opportunity and never looked back. Forensic science has provided me with the most challenging, exciting, and fulfilling career—well beyond any of my expectations. I like the idea of using science to catch the bad guys. Providing justice and closure to victims and their families are the greatest rewards. The intangible benefits of a career in forensic science are priceless.

WENDY'S STORY

Reading *Sherlock Holmes* as a child inspired me to make up stories of villains and murderers to entertain my younger sisters and brother during family outings. My first consulting project as a graduate student in psychology took place at Pennsylvania State Police headquarters in Harrisburg, where I observed dedicated forensic scientists at work in the crime lab. As an industrial-organizational psychologist, I use applied psychology to help improve the workplace. I met Mark when he registered for my M.B.A. class in Human Resource Management. Today, our research involves helping to identify the "people" factors that make forensic technology work better.

can be amplified and matched to a suspect. Invisible biological evidence is now routinely used to solve cases formerly lost in the unsolved cold case file drawer. The 21st century is the century of DNA.

Databases such as CODIS, AFIS, and NIBIN have dramatically increased efficacy in the forensic sciences. However, the education, experience, and commitment of forensic scientists provide the essential human resources needed to apply the new technology to criminal investigations. A recurrent theme throughout the book is the sometimes underappreciated value of this intellectual capital.

The Crime Scene: How Forensic Science Works shows how forensic evidence is processed. It shadows investigators at the crime scene and forensic scientists in the laboratory as they recognize, collect, protect, and analyze evidence. It also provides a realistic job preview of what it is like to be part of the team, giving an overview of the good parts of the job—as well as the challenges. We use a fictional case to show the twists and turns as the case proceeds from first responder to autopsy, from lab work to conviction. Seven appendixes provide extensive resources in the forensic sciences, including lists of references for further reading, accredited colleges and universities in the forensic sciences, and additional Web-based resources. There is also a detailed description of the process for becoming a forensic professional, along with helpful tips and strategies. In addition, a detailed job analysis documents the knowledge, skills, and abilities needed for forensic scientists. Technical documents provide the ILAC G19 2002 guidelines for forensic science laboratories and a summary of the international standard ISO/IEC 17025:2005 general requirements for the competence of testing and calibration laboratories.

Welcome to the world of forensic science!

CHAPTER 1

Crime Scene Situation

Every Contact Leaves Its Trace

—The Locard Principle

"Wherever he steps, whatever he touches, whatever he leaves, even unconsciously, will serve as a silent witness against him. Not only his fingerprints or his foot-prints, but his hair, the fibers from his clothes, the glass he breaks, the tool mark he leaves, the paint he scratches, the blood or semen he deposits or collects. All of these and more, bear mute witness against him. This is evidence that does not forget. It is not confused by the excitement of the moment. It is not absent because human witnesses are. It is factual evidence. Physical evidence cannot be wrong, it cannot perjure itself, it cannot be wholly absent. Only human failure to find it, study and understand it, can diminish its value."

—Professor Edmond Locard, cited in Chisum and Turvey (2000)

The Locard Principle and the Concept of Known and Questioned Evidence

The essence of forensic science is known as the Locard principle, quoted above. A very simplified Locard principle: "You will always leave part of yourself when you are in a room, and you will always take part of the room with you when you leave." An even simpler way to think about the Locard principle: "Every contact leaves its trace." It is up to the forensic scientist to recognize, collect, and protect the evidence, and then produce a meaningful analysis. A forensic scientist must understand the concept of the Locard principle and know the many scientific techniques available at the laboratory.

Let's look at a crime scene. We begin with a brief overview of the process of crime scene analysis. There are a variety of techniques and tools used to visualize and collect all types of evidence. There are no limits as to what constitutes evidence at the crime scene.

The application of the Locard principle is the comparison of *known items* and *questioned items,* Ks and Qs. For example, a fingerprint found at the crime scene is "questioned" because we do not know whose fingerprint it is. The fingerprint could belong to the victim. Or the fingerprint could

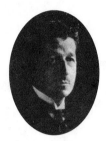

**Edmond Locard
(1877–1966)**

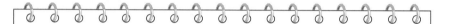

MARK'S STORY

Over the years, our lab investigated serial homicide cases with multiple crime scenes and multiple victims. One particular case stands out. The homicides had been committed over a period of more than 10 years and we had gathered thousands of items of evidence, consisting of both microscopic and macroscopic materials. We had sent hundreds of items of this evidence to the Federal Bureau of Investigation (FBI) laboratory in Washington, D.C. At that time, the FBI was the only lab in the country performing DNA analysis. We had developed an elaborate method of numbering the items of evidence. Frankly, we felt we were the only ones who could understand the relationship between these various pieces of evidence.

Due to the complexity of the case, we felt it necessary to meet with the FBI investigators. A very wise and experienced scientist pulled me aside and said, "Okay kid, bring your evidence over to my lab and we will figure this out." The only thing he carried with him was a black Magic Marker. I proudly started to explain our numbering system, when he interrupted me, saying, "What are the Ks and Qs?" As I explained the first item—the blood of the victim—he took out the Magic Marker and wrote a large K1 on the evidence label. Next he wrote Q1 through Q25 for the 25 blood drops we wanted to compare to K1. It only took him about one hour to classify all the Ks and Qs in this *very complex* case. His simple classification of all the Ks and Qs followed the evidence through the laboratory, to the final report, and into the courtroom. I never forgot this lesson. This basic system of Ks and Qs can help design any laboratory analysis—from the simple to the most complex.

belong to an innocent family member who lives in the house. Or the fingerprint could belong to the perpetrator—the criminal whom investigators wish to catch. A "K," or known item, is a fingerprint obtained from a suspect, so its source is known. Another example is a fingerprint available in a database of fingerprints, taken from known convicted offenders. The whole point of Locard's principle is matching Ks and Qs.

Locard's principle of transfer and comparison of known and questioned items is greatly facilitated by electronic databases, or electronic Ks and Qs. The three major electronic forensic databases are the Combined DNA Index System (CODIS), Automated Fingerprint Identification System (AFIS), and National Integrated Ballistic Information Network (NIBIN). In the United States, these databases are supported by national government agencies. CODIS and AFIS are supported by the FBI, and NIBIN is supported by the Bureau of Alcohol, Tobacco, Firearms and Explosives.

Knowledge of the Locard principle, scientific techniques available at the laboratory, and the comparison of Ks and Qs provide the big picture of how scientists recognize evidence, process a crime scene, and plan laboratory analyses. Newly developed computer databases now compare Ks and Qs, as further described in chapter 17.

Understanding Laboratory Techniques and Laboratory Capacity

A forensic scientist must understand laboratory techniques and capacity when recognizing, collecting, protecting, and submitting evidence for analysis. It is important to know what techniques are available. If one technique is not available in a given laboratory, then it may be possible to send the evidence out to another private or public forensic laboratory. Each forensic laboratory cannot perform all possible forensic techniques that are available; it's just too expensive. For example, mitochondrial DNA analysis is useful for hair shafts and decayed biological materials. But this is a very time-consuming and costly technique that is only done by a few specialized laboratories. This type of evidence can be outsourced to one of the private or public agency mitochondrial DNA laboratories.

In addition, the forensic scientist must also understand the requirements for specific tests. For example, scientists must understand the amount of biological material needed for an analysis. Some analyses are conducted with a drop of saliva the size of a quarter. Others can obtain results from a microscopic or invisible sample. Knowledge of the general

Electronic Databases

CODIS. The Combined DNA Index System (CODIS) consists of unknown DNA profiles (Qs) from crime scenes and known DNA profiles (Ks) from convicted offenders. There are local, state, and national DNA systems that compare known and questioned DNA profiles on a regular schedule. The main concept behind all electronic databases is recidivism. *Recidivism* means that criminals are likely to keep committing crimes even *after* being punished. More than 50 percent of convicted offenders have prior convictions. Recidivism results in at least a 10 percent hit rate in the CODIS system. Hits are reported to local law enforcement with the name of the offender and other criminal history information. The Ks (known convicted offender DNA profiles) are routinely compared electronically with the Qs (unknown DNA profiles developed from crime scenes). These comparisons are done regularly and result in thousands of hits that identify suspects in criminal cases. The hit report is used as a lead that identifies a *possible* suspect. The hit report is then used to obtain a court order to acquire a sample of blood or buccal saliva swab to develop a new DNA profile from the suspect (K), which is then compared to the actual DNA profile (Q) evidence in the case. This is the final quality assurance step in the total process. This final match is used to develop reasonable cause to arrest the suspect for the crime.

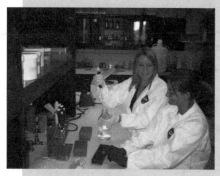

Lab technicians preparing DNA extracts

How many hits can you find in CODIS? Check out CODIS for yourself: *www.fbi.gov/hq/lab/codis/aidedmap.htm.*

How many investigations were aided by CODIS in the state of Virginia? Montana? Which U.S. state has the *most* investigations aided? Which state has the *fewest?*

sensitivities for all forensic analysis lab work is critical when evaluating the evidence in a case. Laboratory analyses can then be planned to maximize information obtained from the evidence.

The forensic scientist must also know the capacity, throughput, or cycle time that is needed, how long it takes for a particular analysis, and

NIBIN. The National Integrated Ballistic Information Network (NIBIN) uses digital photographs of the firing pin and breech mark impressions found on the rear of expended cartridge cases. These unique impressions are formed when the back of the cartridge is pressed against the breech and firing pin when a shot is fired from a weapon. Cartridge extractor marks are also made on the side of the shell casing when the casing is

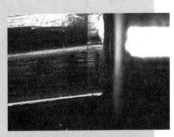

Two bullets viewed from a comparison microscope

ejected from the weapon. In addition to the casing, the projectile is imprinted with lands and grooves that are the mirror image of the unique lands and grooves in the rifled barrel of a gun. All of the microscopic markings can be photographed and placed in NIBIN for comparison. The Ks are images from cartridges and projectiles fired from known weapons. The Qs are casings and projectiles collected at crime scenes. A hit between the Ks and Qs is reported to law enforcement agencies as a lead and is used to obtain a search warrant if needed, in order to obtain the suspected weapon for test firings. The recovered weapon is test fired and the resulting cartridge and projectile (K) is compare to the actual evidence in the case (Q). If there is a match, then the suspect is arrested for the crime.

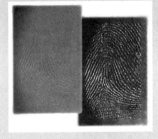

Automated Fingerprint Identification System

AFIS. The Automated Fingerprint Identification System (AFIS) uses electronic records of fingerprints. The Ks (known fingerprints from the 10 print cards taken when suspects are arrested) are compared to Qs (unknown, but identifiable latent fingerprints developed from crime scenes) using imaging and correlation software. The resulting matches are reported as a lead to the appropriate law enforcement agency. As in CODIS, the hit letter is used to request a court order to obtain new fingerprints from the suspect (Ks), which are compared to the latent fingerprints lifted from the crime scene (Qs). The resulting match will be used to develop reasonable cause to arrest the suspect for the crime.

which cases will be selected. For example, if every hair and fiber collected at a crime scene were sent to the lab for comparison, the microscopy section of the laboratory could be overwhelmed for months with just that one case. It is just not feasible to do hundreds or thousands of analyses for each crime that has been committed. The forensic scientist must select the best evidence to process for each case, understanding the realities of the big picture.

Continuous education, involvement in professional organizations, and a network of contacts help a forensic scientist remain effective. Twenty years ago one needed a bachelor's degree to perform forensic analyses. The trend now is to possess a master's degree, particularly for supervisors. Doctoral degrees are becoming increasingly common in all of the forensic disciplines. Scientists stay involved in professional associations and actively develop relationships with colleagues in their discipline. These intangible assets of the laboratory are priceless and often make the difference between an average and excellent laboratory (further described in the Dale and Becker [2005] article entitled "Managing Intellectual Capital" referenced in appendix A).

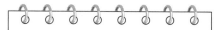

National standards implemented by the Federal Bureau of Investigation, Scientific Working Group on DNA Analyses Methods (SWG-DAM) mandate that forensic supervisors possess an appropriate master's degree in their discipline, with specific courses included in the curriculum (refer to appendixes B and C).

All of the findings and opinions from forensic scientific analyses are subject to a final comparison to the facts of the criminal investigation. How do the opinions generated by the forensic scientist match up to the statements and facts generated by the detectives investigating the crime? Do the pictures of the crime scene support statements from suspects, victims, and witnesses? Can the crime scene be reconstructed to explain the location and relationships of all the evidence in the scene? Are there any discrepancies between the scientific opinions and investigative facts that cannot be explained?

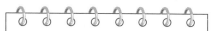

"How often have I said to you that when you have eliminated the impossible, whatever remains, *however improbable*, must be the truth?"

—Sherlock Holmes in *The Sign of the Four* by Sir Arthur Conan Doyle

The forensic scientist must also keep in mind that each and every task will be audited for compliance with the ISO/IEC 17025 accreditation processes *and* challenged in a court of law. Every task performed must be documented as per who performed the task, when it was performed, and the method used. Any human errors must be fully recorded and revealed for all peers, supervisors, administrators, prosecutors, and defense attorneys. Scientists must testify to and document every task that was performed from the crime scene and from the beginning to the end of the laboratory

FIGURE 1.1 *Forensic Scientists Must Know the Big Picture*

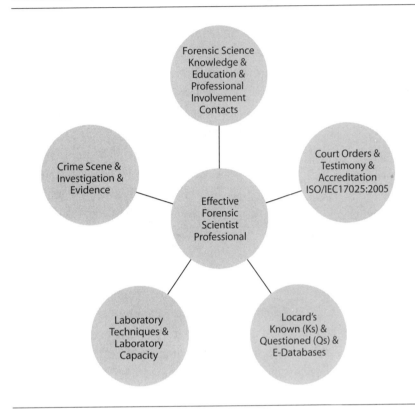

analysis. All work will be vetted by a defense expert who looks for the slightest flaw in the analysis.

Understanding the Big Picture

Forensic laboratories are usually part of a police agency, such as a township, city, county, state, or federal law enforcement agencies. A forensic scientist may work alone or in a team of professionals to process a crime scene. In a small police department, one person may perform all crime scene tasks. Large departments have specialists that work together as a team.

All laboratories must have quality systems in place to be sure that they consistently produce valid results. ISO/IEC 17025:2005 is the main standard used by testing and calibration laboratories. There are two main sections involved, management requirements and technical requirements. The management requirements are concerned with the efficient operation and effectiveness of quality management systems within the laboratory.

The technical requirements are concerned with the competence of staff, methodology and the testing and calibration of equipment. Accreditation has to do with maintaining these quality standards at all times (refer to Appendix F, Accreditation Standards).

In most departments, sworn police officers are crime scene technicians. Officers interested in forensics are selected for entry-level positions after an evaluation of their experience and education, and move up to positions of more responsibility and expertise. Civilian personnel provide assistance for the full-time sworn crime scene officer. Some police departments have partially or completely civilianized the crime scene function.

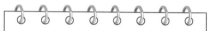

An example of a forensic laboratory mission statement: "The mission of the forensic lab is to apply the best science to the best evidence in a timely manner with no errors."

Did you know that the home residence is the most common crime scene? For example, a burglary can quickly escalate into a violent crime if the homeowner confronts the intruder. The intruder may panic and attack the owner while trying to get away. A violent crime investigation, such as a homicide, may develop more than one crime scene. For example, there might be a residence, an automobile, an autopsied body, and an outside area where the body was found. All of these venues are considered separate crime scenes and must be processed individually, in the context of the total criminal investigation.

All evidence that places the suspect in the residence and that supports the theory of how the crime occurred will be collected at the residence. The suspect's vehicle will be processed for any evidence that is unique to the residence or victim of the homicide. The victim's body will be processed for any evidence that is unique to the suspect, residence, or vehicle, in addition to determining the cause of death.

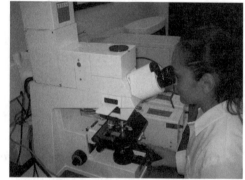

Scientist using microscope to recognize evidence

The forensic scientist must be aware of one caveat that lessens the importance of the evidence in all cases: If the victim and suspect have had previous encounters or relationships, the significance of the Locard principle will be diminished or even nullified. For example, if the victim and suspect lived together, the transfer of fibers, hairs, or fingerprints will be insignificant in many instances. There are exceptions. A bloody fingerprint from the suspect on a murder weapon places the weapon in the hand of the suspect. A bloody fingerprint from the suspect made from the victim's blood is a very probative item of evidence, even if the suspect had prior access to the residence. These facts are very significant, even when victim and suspect lived together or had prior contact.

The fictional "Laura Lake" story beginning at the end of this chapter follows a team of crime scene personnel, forensic experts, and members of law enforcement agencies as they work to solve a murder case. As the story progresses throughout the book, it outlines the process of crime scene investigation, laboratory analyses, and courtroom testimony for the Laura Lake homicide. The Crime Scene Process Flow Chart (centerpiece) details the sequential steps of the investigation. There is an administrative, technical, and quality assurance review of all major steps of the process. Any outcomes that do not meet quality standards will be reviewed and reanalyzed until they are in concordance with all methods and policies.

Laura Lake Residence, 159 Walnut Street, Metroland, New York

CRIME SCENE

Local businessperson Laura Lake has operated a successful jewelry business in Metroland, New York, with her family for over 20 years. Laura wants to open new stores and expand Lake Jewelry to neighboring communities to provide more opportunities for family members. Laura was recently given a small business award by the area chamber of commerce because of Lake Jewelry's generous support for local charities. As part of the award ceremony, Metroland News interviewed Laura, providing recognition for her very successful family business.

Laura lives in the Metroland suburbs. Most residents leave for work early in the morning and the suburban neighborhood is relatively deserted during the day. Laura is a hard worker and would normally be at work, but today she is meeting with a new landscaper who left a flyer in her door. She usually researches contractors thoroughly but was desperate to get some yard work done.

Lake's neighbor, Betty Smith, is outside picking up the paper from her driveway, when she hears loud, unusual noises coming from the Lakes' home. She calls 911, and emergency technician Mary Marcel is the first one on the scene. Mary arrives driving the ambulance. Patrol Officer Barry Lasker is the next to arrive in his patrol car.

First responders establish the scene as safe and provide care for any victims found at the scene. Both Barry and Mary have little experience with criminal cases and no experience with a homicide. Mary's mission is to provide lifesaving support to victims as soon as possible at the risk of compromising or destroying any evidence. She goes right to Laura Lake, administers CPR, and uses a portable defibrillator. In her rush, she accidentally steps in some blood. Mary knows that she could destroy some of the evidence but she also knows that a live victim is better than a dead one.

CHAPTER 2

First Responder

The Team Approach

Police, fire, and emergency medical technicians work as a team at the scene of a crime. Creating teams from multiple agencies may appear difficult or even impossible at times; however, these emergency response agencies train together so that they can complement one another's activities. Whether responding to the scene of a crime, fire, or accident, all share a common goal: to provide the best emergency service to the community. Establishing professional relationships between agencies and personnel at the scene is the key to providing

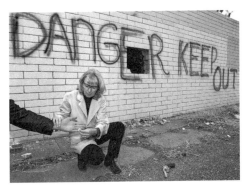

An emergency response team at the scene.

the most efficient and highest quality response to the emergency. It takes extensive training in the team approach to establish a coordinated response to emergencies.

Most forensic crime laboratories are located within a law enforcement agency. Law enforcement agencies are paramilitary organizations that operate in a command-and-control environment. Simply stated, this means that when the police investigate a crime, they are in total charge from when they arrive to when they release the scene. It is paramount that police establish the safety of all individuals and the integrity of the evidence.

The paramilitary nature of law enforcement means that there are specific lines of supervision, spans of control, and responsibilities for assignments. For example, all personnel report to only one supervisor. There are often "hard dates" when tasks must be completed. For example, interviews may be needed to present findings to a grand jury within a certain deadline. Laboratory reports may also be needed for court proceedings. All personnel at the crime scene have specific tasks to complete in a timely manner with no errors. This environment of supervision, control, tasks, and accountability can be very stressful. Forensic scientists are trained to perform at a high level that exceeds performance expectations.

The first police officer at the scene takes charge of the incident. She must identify herself as a police officer and clearly state her role and responsibilities to others. Upon evaluating the incident, the officer notifies supervisors and determines if additional assistance from other units or crime scene personnel is needed. She must make notifications in a timely manner, using proper protocol. She may request additional personnel from fire or medical teams. Safety is the priority at the scene.

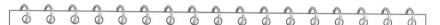

New York State has hundreds of police agencies and 62 district attorneys. They meet regularly with the forensic laboratories to review cases in preparation for trial. The New York State District Attorney's Association has requested a training program to standardize the *documentation* of tasks performed at the scene to provide a logical and sequential series of events that would maximize the efficiency of the investigation and collection of evidence. Ultimately, it is the district attorney who has the responsibility to present the chronological description of the tasks performed at the scene to the jury. Presentation to the jury involves direct testimony, documents, and evidence. A training program to standardize and document the tasks at a crime scene facilitates the prosecutor's role in a criminal trial. The district attorneys emphasized that the most important factor in a criminal investigation is note taking. The investigator must take copious and accurate notes of all things he does, sees, and hears, in chronological order, with no errors.

The first police officer, firefighter, or medical personnel to arrive at the scene of the crime may be perceived as the first responder. However, in most cases there are other individuals who actually were the first to arrive on the scene, and who initially *requested* that police, fire, or medical personnel respond. These individuals could be a neighbor of the victim, who noticed that the newspaper and mail had not been picked up for days. The neighbor or friend might have taken the next step to check on the acquaintance, and noticed that no one came to the door. They possess valuable information critical to the criminal investigation. Infrequently, the fire, police, or medical personnel are the first on the scene. They must be careful not to compromise one another's responsibilities at the scene.

When the police officer receives a call over the radio to respond to a crime scene, there is a logical sequence of events that must be followed to ensure everyone's safety and the proper investigation of the incident. The incident may have begun as a minor dispute between family members and developed into a serious assault or even a homicide. The police officer must treat all responses the same way, anticipating that the case will proceed to trial and be subjected to the policies and procedures of the criminal justice system.

The RESPOND Protocol

In response to requests from the District Attorney's Association, the New York State Police worked with agencies across the state to develop a concise training program for first responders, to standardize documentation and the steps taken at a crime scene in *any* jurisdiction across the state. That program is the following:

- **R** RESPOND
- **E** EVALUATE
- **S** SECURE
- **P** PROTECT
- **O** OBSERVE
- **N** NOTIFY
- **D** DOCUMENT

These elements are general tasks that are part of the first responder protocol nationwide.

Respond

First responders act in response to all crimes, possible break-ins, and burglaries and must assume that the suspect is still in the residence. Observations are made even on the way to the crime scene. For example, the suspect may be fleeing and pass the first responder on the same roadway. First responders must stay alert and make mental notes. Suspicious vehicles and pedestrians tend to avoid marked patrol vehicles, but first responders should try to take note of the make, model, color, and license plates of these vehicles as well as any pedestrian descriptions. A tape recorder can serve as an archive for first responder observations and notes can be transcribed later that day. Notes are written as contemporaneously with the observation as possible. These notes will be leads for police to follow up on after the initial response.

Safety is a priority for the police officer, complainant, witnesses, and any bystanders. There may be an armed suspect still in the residence or nearby. Assistance of special units may be needed to secure the safety of the scene. There could be chemical, electrical, or fire hazards that need to be stabilized before the scene is processed. Personal protective equipment may be necessary to protect responders from chemical, biological, or radiological pathogens. All personnel must have the protective equipment needed before entering the scene.

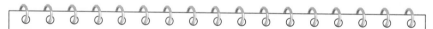

Think about this: Would you be able to document every detail about everything you did, saw, and heard yesterday without any errors? Would you be able to testify in court from these notes, one or two years from now?

Evaluate

First responders next determine what type of crime has occurred. The crime could be a lesser offense like a burglary, a more serious assault, or even a homicide. Crime scene personnel consult closely with investigating detectives and the prosecutor to define the offenses. Assistance may be needed from specialized units from the police department, emergency medical technicians, or fire department. Witnesses, victims, and bystanders must be interviewed only after the scene is secure and no additional assistance is needed from medical or fire personnel. Assistance may be needed to interview a large number of witnesses. These witnesses may be difficult to locate after they leave the scene.

Secure

First responders establish an inner and outer perimeter. The inner perimeter is only for crime scene personnel. The outer perimeter is for other investigative personnel. It must be clearly established who is authorized within each perimeter zone. An attendance log documents *who* is within these zones and *when*.

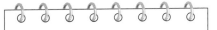

First responders must adhere to Locard's principle, "Every contact leaves a trace." It is essential not to contaminate the scene *in any way.*

Protect

Crime scene personnel must protect the scene from all factors that degrade or affect the integrity of the evidence. The crime scene area must be protected from the weather. If the scene is outside, then rain, wind, or snow may affect footprints or blood spatter. Animals, wild or domestic, may destroy or scatter human remains. Unnecessary traffic from humans or vehicles will create the potential for contamination and loss of evidence. Temperature may affect the composition of any liquids, foodstuffs, or plumbing in a residence.

Observe

Observations and senses are critical as a first responder. Responding personnel will ask the witness to describe everything seen and heard. This takes a lot of practice. Often the scene is chaotic at this stage with a victim who is injured and family members who are present. Emotions run high. The first responder is expected to present a demeanor of stability and calm. It takes practice, training, and strong mentor relationships from experienced professionals.

It is helpful for first responders to use checklists that describe their responsibilities. Police are

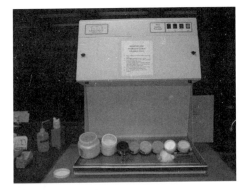

Fingerprint powders

also human, and are subject to human error. The best way to learn these skills is through the investigation of lesser offenses, such as larceny and burglary. The skills learned through lesser offenses are exactly the same as those used in major cases.

Notify

First responders must notify numerous supervisors, support units, and agencies in a timely manner. Notifications are clear, concise, and categorical, not "I *think* this is what is going on," or "I am not quite sure." They must provide a clear description of what has taken place so that supervisors can determine if more resources are needed. All radio and electronic communications that have transpired will be used to investigate the case and will ultimately be provided to the prosecutor and defense. First responders are called to testify in court, under oath, and must account for all actions that they have taken.

At the very least, and depending on the agency's policies and procedures, the following people will be notified:

- Supervisors
- Medical examiner
- District attorney
- Emergency medical technicians
- Fire department
- Other law enforcement agencies
- Next of kin

Document

One of the most difficult parts of responding to the crime scene is the documentation of observations. Software and computers are available to help perform this task, but even the most sophisticated technology is only as good as the first responder's basic ability to document observations. Notes must be accurate and taken at the same time that the observation was made. Time cannot be wasted when updating documentation. Completing tasks in a prearranged, sequential order is essential. Documentation can be kept as simple as possible. This task is made more complex when more than one individual or agency is processing the scene.

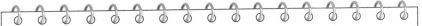

Documentation includes basic facts, such as time of call, time of arrival, a basic sketch of the scene, the weather, the temperature, doors open, doors locked, mode of entry, mode of exit, lights on, lights off, thermostat setting, etc.

A chronological and concise narrative of what is seen and what has been done is essential and difficult. This requires adequate writing and computer skills. Responders become known for their report writing and ability to be articulate to peers, supervisors, prosecutors, and juries. Communication must be intelligible. All information from the first responder will be turned over to the detective and crime scene team. Ultimately, first responders testify in court to their notes.

First responders provide the following documentation:

- Attendance log
  - Inner perimeter
  - Outer perimeter
- Narrative of everything done,
  seen, and heard
- Witness statements

At this point, the responsibilities and tasks of the first responder have ended and the situation is stable. Authority is transferred to the professional team with specialized skills that will process the crime scene.

Frequently Asked Questions

Q: *Are most first responders trained police officers, firefighters, or emergency medical technicians?*

A: First responder personnel represent all three professions. Fire and EMT personnel are mainly concerned with the safety and medical attention of victims. The fire department fights fires and responds to a variety of incidents similar to the police. However, when it is clear that a crime has been committed, the scene is turned over to police personnel.

Q: *What is the most difficult task for the first responder?*

A: The first responder has many difficult tasks including making accurate observations and taking good notes. One of the most difficult tasks of the first responder is to maintain calm, control the situation, and perform responsibilities without error.

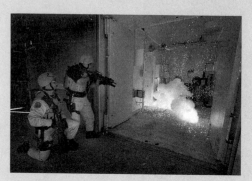

First responders

LAURA LAKE ATTENDANCE LOG
Laura Lake Residence, 159 Walnut Street,
Metroland, New York

Metroland Police Department
Crime Scene Attendance Log
Form CSU #1

Location	Victim	Precinct	Established/ Maintained By	Case Number	Perimeter
Address: 159 Walnut Street, Metroland, New York 12345-6789	Laura Lake	22	Patrol Officer Barry Lasker	A492	Inner perimeter

Date	Name	Agency	Time In	Time Out	Authorized to Enter? Y/N
April 1, 2010	Mary Marcel, EMT	Metroland EMT	1100 hours	1430 hours	Y
April 1, 2010	Barry Lasker, Patrol Officer	Metroland PD	1130 hours	2300 hours	Y
April 1, 2010	Daniel Escobar, Detective Lieutenant	Metroland PD	1300 hours	2305 hours	Y
April 1, 2010	Betty Smith	Neighbor	1145 hours	1245 hours	N

CHAPTER 3

Team Responsibilities at the Crime Scene

The crime scene team leader determines the resources needed to process the crime scene after evaluating the information provided by the first officer on the scene. Resources are assigned commensurate with the magnitude of the crime and availability of personnel. The responding officer or a crime scene technician may process a minor incident, such as a burglary, alone. For major cases, a small department may ask for assistance from a neighboring city or state's crime scene unit. Assignments are made for the following:

- Crime scene team leader
- Photographer
- Sketch preparer
- Evidence custodian
- Evidence recovery team
- Additional specialists, as needed

Crime Scene Team Leader

The crime scene team leader assumes control of the scene from the beginning to the end of the process. The main concern of the crime scene team leader is the *safety and security* of the scene. There can be no injuries or security concerns at the crime scene location. Once the safety and security of the scene are established, the crime scene team leader will perform an initial

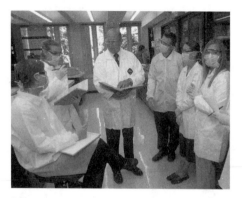

Crime scene team

walk-through to evaluate potential evidence and will start documenting what she does, hears, and sees. A mechanism for communication will be established between forensic and investigative personnel. Coordination with other units and agencies will be maintained. The crime scene team leader will also ensure that all equipment and consumable supplies are available to the crime scene team. The crime scene team leader is ultimately responsible for the inventory, proper collection, packaging, labeling (bagging and tagging), and chain of custody for all evidence removed from the scene.

The last responsibility of the crime scene team leader is to release the scene. This decision is critical, as the team may not have another opportunity to return to the scene and gather more evidence. Team members have one chance to do it right. In addition, some items of evidence may be noxious or in the process of degradation; these must be transported to the laboratory quickly.

Photographer

When possible, one person is assigned responsibly for taking all photographs. The photographer is one of the most important members of the team. Photographs taken at the crime scene will be viewed by everyone who has a need to know about the case. They will be the subject of subpoenas and court orders. The photographs will be the only way to view the crime scene after it is released, and they must thoroughly and with the utmost detail describe all aspects of the crime scene.

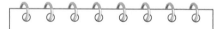

Experienced crime scene personnel know that their goal is to *handle the evidence once and do it right*. That simple statement is the essence of quality assurance for the total forensic process.

The photographer must photograph the entire area of the crime scene before any personnel enter. At this point, the crime scene is pristine, except for the first responders, EMTs, fire personnel, victims, and any other activity that can be confirmed as having taken place after the incident. The entire area must be photographed before the scene is processed. All victims must be photographed, along with their injuries.

Live victims' injuries will heal and will not be visible later in court. The crowd and any vehicles in the surrounding area must be photographed completely. There may be other witnesses that emerge later in the case. The suspect may be in the crowd as a bystander. The entire scene is photographed using overall, medium, and close-up lenses, and using measurement scales. The scale, preferably with a color gradient, is critical. The date, time, and identification of the photographer should be imprinted in all digital files and negatives.

A record of all photographs must be prepared and constantly updated. The backs of all photographs will also be marked to correspond with all information in the photograph record. It is common to have hundreds of photographs taken in a criminal investigation. Accurate record keeping is critical for the establishment of

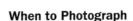

When to Photograph

When in doubt, take a photograph! It may be the only opportunity to capture an image of a person, place, or thing at the crime scene.

proper files in anticipation of courtroom testimony. The photographs of destroyed latent prints or footprint impressions are also treated as evidence. These photographs are stored with the same security, seals, and chain of custody as other tangible items of evidence.

Sketch Preparer

A sketch or diagram is used to show the location of all evidence, victim(s), and other probative information of the crime scene, such as important distance and size relationships. The sketch must have basic points of reference, such as orientation to the north and proper scale. All items of evidence are indicated on the diagram and the same nomenclature must be used to mark the evidence. All exterior buildings, roads, telephone poles, interior rooms, and furnishings must be placed in the diagram. Specific areas must have labels or nomenclature. All team members must use the same names for these designated areas. The sketch preparer may need assistance in preparing the sketch, such as help making measurements and taking notes. All personnel assisting in the preparation of the sketch must be listed. Technology has impacted this area of crime scene processing. Laser measuring tools and survey equipment complemented with computer applications are very useful for certain crime scene applications.

Evidence Custodian

The evidence custodian or recorder is one of the most important team members at the crime scene. The labeling of evidence in a clear and uniform manner is difficult, particularly when there is more than one scene. Complications may also arise when additional evidence is collected at a later date and submitted to the laboratory for analysis. Evidence numbers must be unique for each particular item of evidence. The evidence custodian must coordinate closely with the sketch preparer to ensure that the evidence labels and sketch are in perfect agreement. An accurate inventory and location of all items of evidence must be established and maintained from the initial collection, through laboratory analyses, courtroom presentation, and finally, in long-term storage, in anticipation of any appeals. Any errors in these tasks can prove to be catastrophic later in the laboratory or courtroom presentations.

The evidence custodian also maintains the chain of custody for all items of evidence. This task can become very complex when there are a large number of items being tracked from multiple locations. The chain of custody consists of three main components: authorized persons, designated locations, and dates and times of evidence transfers. Evidence is transferred between authorized persons (P to P), authorized persons to designated locations (P to L), or designated locations to authorized persons (L to P). These transactions must be dated, with time listed if deemed necessary. The transactions for the chain of custody must also be documented with initials or signature of authorized personnel at the time of the transaction.

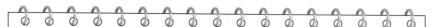

Chain of Custody

The evidence custodian cannot wait until the end of the day or during a break to document the chain of custody. The chain of custody documentation must be performed when the transaction occurs between authorized people and locations. Any breaks in the chain of custody may result in the item of evidence being excluded from trial proceedings.

Evidence Recovery Team

The actual collection of evidence consists of several sequential components performed by one person or a team. The first step is the recognition of the evidence, followed by the collection, and then protection against degradation, loss, and contamination. There is only one chance to collect the evidence and items cannot be missed. Therefore, crime scene technicians collect many items, even though they are not sure initially of the value of all of the items. They do not want to eliminate any items at this early stage of the investigation.

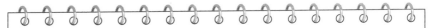

Bagging and Tagging

Some agencies call this step "bagging and tagging." When new officers first start going to crime scenes, it is very difficult to assess the scene and actually recognize the evidence needed to support the investigation of the crime. Has anything been missed? Crime scene technicians can seldom go back to reprocess the scene.

Recognition of some evidence can be accomplished with natural light when the items are large enough to see with the naked eye. There are also chemical enhancements (i.e., luminol) that show a color change when exposed to the iron in blood. Superglue fuming will enhance latent fingerprints that are not visible. Trace evidence that resulted from a person or tool's contact with a surface may be invisible to the naked eye. Common contact surfaces such as keyboards, light switches, phones, and door handles may contain trace amounts of DNA from human biological materials. It is common to obtain a full DNA profile from a contact surface. Experienced crime scene personnel know where to look and how to collect contact evidence. There are general guidelines used by evidence recovery teams for all types of evidence. These procedures will be explained in further detail in chapters 4 through 10.

All evidence must be fully photographed after recognition and before collection. The sketch preparer must be advised of the location. The best method for collection must be determined. Most agencies use disposable forceps to collect items of evidence; items are then placed in standardized sterile evidence containers. At a minimum, the containers must be marked with the agency case number, item number, who collected the item, and when the item was collected. The item container is then sealed to protect against loss, and the seal is dated and initialed. All items are packaged separately to protect against cross-contamination. Biological items are dried and stored in refrigeration to protect against biodegradation.

Safety from bloodborne pathogens is critical for all personnel who process evidence. In the United States, all police agencies comply with the Occupational Safety and Health Administration (OSHA) Bloodborne Pathogens Standard 1910.1030, that protects personnel through the use of the proper personal protective equipment.

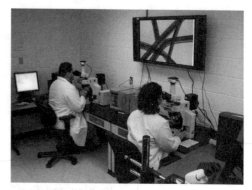

Evidence recovery team

Specialists

It is sometimes necessary to bring in expertise from other public laboratories, industry, the academic community, or private scientific laboratories. Examples of specialty assistance include the following:

- Medical examiner/coroner
- Odontologist
- Anthropologist
- Entomologist
- Blood pattern analyst
- Geologist
- Surveyor
- Engineer
- Bomb technician
- Forensic scientist
- Forensic artist

Frequently Asked Questions

Q: *What is the difference between civilian and sworn personnel?*

A: Federal, state, and local laws define law enforcement officers (sworn personnel) as individuals who ordinarily carry a firearm and a badge, have full arrest powers, and are paid from government funds set aside specifically for law enforcement. Civilian employees include personnel such as forensic scientists, crime analysts, mechanics, radio dispatchers, and other full-time employees of the agency.

Q: *Is it normal for civilian and sworn personnel to work side by side at a crime scene?*

A: Yes, civilian and sworn personnel work very closely together in many ways. Civilian personnel provide support for many police functions.

Q: *Are the roles clearly defined among all personnel responsible for processing a crime scene?*

A: Yes, they are clearly defined. In a lesser offense, such as a burglary, all of the responsibilities may be performed by only one individual.

Q: *What laws provide the authority of the medical examiner?*

A: In most states, local or county law provides the authority for the medical examiner to take control of a body at a crime scene. The relationship between the medical examiner, police department, and crime scene unit is critical. There may be instances in which the death is accidental and no crime has been committed. These decisions are made very early in an investigation and may require an autopsy to confirm the cause of death.

CRIME SCENE

Laura Lake Residence, 159 Walnut Street, Metroland, New York

Olivia Johns, forensic scientist supervisor, has worked in the lab for 10 years. She was appointed a position at the forensic science lab after taking the civil service exam and passing the rigorous entry requirements. She has always loved science and has an undergraduate degree in biology from State University. Olivia earned a master's degree in forensic molecular biology while attending school part-time, taking classes at night after working all day at the lab. Olivia does not routinely respond to crime scenes, but the Laura Lake homicide case has received a lot of local media attention. Olivia knows that when forensic scientists in the laboratory work closely with the crime scene technicians at the scene, analyses are more efficient at the laboratory.

Olivia's hard work has paid off and she has accomplished the career goal she set for herself in high school—to be a forensic supervisor who manages major crime forensic laboratory analyses. In her job she feels the pressure from prosecutors, law enforcement, and even family members of victims to analyze all items of evidence with all possible scientific techniques available. Her laboratory has recently hired new forensic technicians, but the lab does not have the resources to analyze all items of evidence collected at the crime scene. Olivia must make intelligent decisions to work efficiently and provide a report in a timely fashion for court.

Olivia is the crime scene team leader for the Laura Lake homicide. She will take control of the scene and work very closely with John Goodspeed, crime scene technician 1, and Dr. Ali Kumar, medical examiner. The medical examiner, or coroner in most jurisdictions, is by law in charge of the body at the crime scene. This means that the body cannot be moved

(continued)

CRIME SCENE

(continued)

in any way until the victim has been examined and declared dead by the medical examiner.

The medical examiner, Metroland Police Department, and crime scene personnel work very closely together as a team for the total crime scene process, laboratory examinations, and courtroom presentations. First responder Barry Lasker and EMT Mary Marcel will update all responding personnel and will then disengage from the crime scene.

The basic responsibilities of all personnel at the scene are also closely coordinated with investigative personnel. Detective Lieutenant Daniel Escobar will also periodically receive an update of the crime scene processing from Olivia Johns. Olivia Johns and John Goodspeed will work as a team to process this crime scene. They realize that Laura Lake was a well-known businesswoman in the community. This case will receive a great deal of attention in the media.

CHAPTER 4

Basic Principles of Evidence Collection, Preservation, and Documentation

C rime scene processing involves a sequential order of tasks, performed by a variety of people, from one or more agencies. The crime scene team leader has overall responsibility for management of the total process. This chapter describes the overall "big picture" of the process and the tasks needed to collect, preserve, and document evidence.

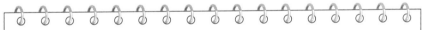

The American Society of Crime Laboratory Directors/Laboratory Accreditation Board (ASCLD/LAB) provides very specific criteria for handling evidence. The ASCLD/LAB program recently designated crime scene processing as a specific forensic discipline. ASCLD/LAB's accreditation process requires that forensic laboratories have policies and procedures that recognize, collect, and protect evidence from degradation, loss, and contamination.

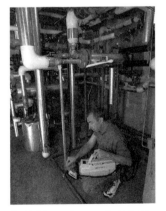

Portable swipe analysis tool

Preparation

Preparation is key to safe and efficient crime scene processing. Medical assistance may be needed, so resources from the local fire and ambulance teams should be on standby. Close relationships with these support agencies is well established during regular interagency meetings and drills. The crime scene team leader considers the safety of personnel and the supplies needed to process the scene.

The crime scene must be processed in a timely manner. Criteria such as time required and the conditions at the crime scene are used to estimate resources needed. Communication and food are priorities for the crime scene unit. Personnel could be at the site for several days, a week, or more. Some agencies have specially designed vehicles that provide support at the site of the crime scene. Inclement weather and crime scenes that are outdoors will require weatherproof clothing and equipment for all personnel. Fast and reliable communication between all team members is essential for successful crime scene processing. Departments routinely use two-way radios, cell and satellite phones, and Internet connectivity, for audio, video, and email. The team may need emergency power, lighting assistance, and shelter.

Perimeter security may be provided by support agencies to allow crime scene personnel to focus on their specific crime scene processing tasks. The crime scene team leader is responsible for assembling all tools needed to collect evidence and document the evidence collection process. All materials are assembled beforehand, including forms (hard copy and computer) and tools needed for the collection of evidence, such as forceps, scalpels, bags, and containers.

Even at this early stage, crime scene personnel work closely with the district attorney to consider legal issues with regard to the search. Legal issues are discussed in more detail in chapter 16. All tasks performed at the scene will be closely reviewed in a hearing or criminal proceeding. The team follows all legal policies and procedures used to collect the evidence in a proper manner. This prevents items of evidence from being excluded in subsequent legal proceedings. For example, a search warrant may be needed to authorize the search of a specific area for specific items. The team does not want to extend the search beyond the limits set in the search warrant.

The crime scene team leader briefs all participants at the crime scene with the overall scope and details of the search. All individuals are assigned specific responsibilities. These assignments must be properly matched to the knowledge, skills, and abilities of the person. Crime scenes that are large or involve multiple locations may require two or more teams. One large scene may require two or more shifts to process the scene in a timely manner. The addition of shifts and multiple teams will add significant administrative responsibilities to the crime scene team leader.

Frequent communication between crime scene personnel, detectives, laboratory forensic scientists, the district attorney, medical examiner, fire department, emergency medical teams, and other support agencies is critical. One individual must be assigned as the contact for all communication. This individual is usually a senior detective with experience in the investigation of a particular type of crime. The senior detective will make assignments for obtaining statements or obtaining other information relative to the investigation. The senior detective, through experience, will recognize correlations between evidence, statements, and laboratory analyses. These "leads" will be identified and assigned to other detectives or forensic scientists to include or exclude from the investigation. Computer programs (data mining software, timelines, etc.) have been applied to this process, with limited success. Having experienced detectives working directly with the crime scene team and the laboratory is the most effective way to solve criminal investigations efficiently. If the detective works separately from

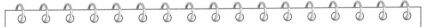

Crime scene tasks can be thought of as part of a complete business process. The crime laboratory is the factory, albeit a very complex suite of technology processes, that applies science to evidence to obtain value or information for use in the criminal trial. The evidence is the raw material, coming into the lab. Rework costs time and money. The total process has less waste if there is a very close relationship between the crime scene (raw materials) and the lab.

As an example, there are many items of evidence submitted to the lab early in the investigative process. Many of these items are excluded from analysis once the investigation begins. A theory develops concerning how the crime was committed. Timely and accurate information sharing between all members of the crime scene/investigative team will eliminate unneeded analysis of items. This allows laboratory resources to be used for other cases and to analyze the maximum amount of probative items of evidence.

the crime scene and forensic personnel, then the investigation will not proceed in the most efficient manner.

Approaching the Scene

All members of the team are alert for discarded criminal evidence on their approach, as the route may have been used by criminals as they fled the scene. Crime scene team members make mental notes and "think aloud" or transcribe notes to others while traveling to the scene. At the same time, the team must be sure to drive to the scene safely.

Securing and Protecting the Scene

The scene must be made secure and be protected at all times. Conversely, the team must determine the extent to which the scene has not been protected. All first responders must be interviewed and their notes must be obtained for inclusion in the case file. Information must be gathered from individuals who entered the scene and have knowledge of its original condition. The team establishes an attendance log; it must be up-to-date and complete, and must indicate individuals who are approved or denied entry to the crime scene.

Initiating a Preliminary Survey—The Initial Walk-Through

The next step is developing a plan to search the total crime scene. The team starts with a cautious walk-through, using the absolute minimum of personnel. A recording device may be used for the narrative to be written later. Alternatively, one individual is designated as the recorder for official notes. The scene is photographed in general along with all major items of evidence. The notes and photographs will be used to describe and explain the scene to other personnel. A log documents all photographs taken at the scene. The limits of the internal perimeter of the scene are determined by starting small and working outward, adding distinct boundaries to the new perimeters. New attendance logs are correlated with the time and date to the proper perimeters. It is critical to document personnel in the scene as potential sources of contamination. Obvious items of evidence are identified and protected. The team must remain objective and serve as fact finders at this stage of the investigation. It is important that team members keep an open mind and not try to solve the crime on the first walk-through of the scene.

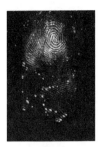

Fingerprint processed with superglue

Evaluating Physical Evidence Possibilities

The scene is evaluated for all possible types of physical evidence. Based on their preliminary walk-through, the team considers what types of evidence are most likely to be found for this type of crime. Was there a murder? Was an assault weapon used by the suspect? The team concentrates first on the most fragile types of evidence. Bacteria will immediately start to degrade biological evidence, such as blood and DNA. This type of evidence must be dried, refrigerated, and taken to the laboratory as soon as possible to reduce the effects of biodegradation. The team focuses on the obvious items in plain view, progressing to out-of-view locations or hidden items. Some items or even the victim may have been moved, purposely by the suspect or inadvertently by responding personnel. The whole scene may have been set up by the suspect to simulate a certain type of accident to hide the fact that a criminal act has taken place. All members of the crime scene team work together to evaluate the scene for this evidence.

Preparing Narrative Description

The narrative description of the scene must accurately portray all of the evidence and the special relationships between the evidence, relevant to the crime. The narrative description is used as a reference for individuals who are not able to view the scene in person. Narratives also serve archival purposes, whether the crime scene is a residence, vehicle, or outside area. The material in the narrative moves from the general to the specific, and it is supplemented with photographs and diagrams.

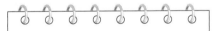

The narrative must provide a chronological description of who did what, when, where, and why. All references to other documents and photographs are included in the narrative description.

Good narratives require good writing skills. Team members must have a solid command of basic writing skills. They must anticipate questions that will be asked by prosecutors, senior command officers, and forensic scientists. No detail is too small to include. Technology including electronic forms, computers, and video cameras with audio can be used to aid the walk-through narrative. Digital records, like hard copy records, must be archived. When possible, one person is designated to write the narrative description.

Depicting the Scene Photographically

Use of photography is one of the most important tasks performed at the crime scene. Other detectives and forensic scientists will ultimately evaluate the theory of how the crime was committed, assisted by photographs. Photographs are not taken randomly. A plan to photograph the scene is developed, using a system that includes a photograph record. All photos must be accounted for and made a part of the official investigative record. The photographs must begin with the overall scene and then progress to individual rooms, compartments, and then items of evidence. Certified photographic measurement scales (color, black and white, and size) are needed for all photographs. All evidence must be photographed in place before being moved or changed in any way. The methods of collection, packaging, seals, and labels used on all items of evidence are photographed. These photographs will support the accurate documentation of the evidence inventory collected and removed from the scene.

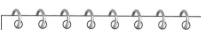

Evidence integrity is compromised in a trial if there is not a proper photographic record of the evidence collection process.

Photographs are also taken in areas adjacent to the crime scene, to place the scene in the proper perspective. This may include other rooms and buildings. Points of entry and exit need to be documented and examined for pry marks and other trace evidence left by the suspect, such as hair, fibers, blood, or fingerprints. The photographer correlates all photographs with maps, blueprints, security cameras, aerial photography, and satellite imaging to identify additional information, such as people, vehicles, or other landmarks. Photographs should be taken at eye level, if possible, or at the level that would be observed in a normal view. The photographer should take pictures of all fragile items of evidence from multiple vantage positions if there is a possibility that the evidence may be compromised or lost during the collection process.

Preparing a Diagram or Sketch of the Scene

A rough sketch is drawn during the preliminary walk-through of the scene. This rudimentary sketch is not drawn to scale, but is used to record the location of any important items of evidence and victims. The sketch is

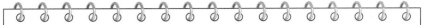

It is possible to lose or destroy a latent print, tool mark, or shoe print during normal processing and lifting of these items. If lost, the photograph will serve as the item of evidence for comparison to known controls. All photographs must be referenced to all diagrams, narratives, and witness and victim statements. Matching of photographs with the total crime scene process, and the statements of victims and suspects, are valuable tools for detectives. Any statements that do not precisely correspond with the appropriate photographs will need to be resolved by more interviews with victims, suspects, and witnesses and correlated with other evidence.

The crime scene process itself must have no bias—no stake in the outcome of the investigation.

coordinated with the photographs. The rough sketch would include at least the following:

- Specific location
- Lighting conditions
- Date
- Scale or scale disclaimer
- Time
- Compass orientation
- Case identifier
- Evidence
- Preparer/assistants
- Measurements
- Weather conditions
- Key or legend

It is very important that all evidence numbers on the sketch are correlated with the same number designations on the evidence log. The rough sketch, in most instances, will be used as a model to prepare a detailed scale diagram of the scene. Some police agencies assign individuals with artistic, architectural, or draftsman expertise to work with the crime scene personnel to develop the final sketch of the scene. There are computer-aided design (CAD) programs and surveying equipment that can be used to prepare crime scene diagrams. These computer programs use electronic records and templates from house or roadway blueprints to prepare a very accurate crime scene diagram.

Conducting a Detailed Search and Collecting Physical Evidence

Now the evidence must be recognized, collected, and protected against loss, degradation, and contamination. A grid, strip, or circle search pattern is used to search in specific areas, proceeding from the general to the specific and including all types of evidence. **The key is to do it once and do it right the first time.** All items are photographed before and after collection and the correct notations are entered in the photograph record. The location of all items of evidence is marked on the crime scene diagram.

Latent fingerprints are one of the most important types of physical evidence, because of their ability to place an individual at the scene. Latent fingerprints require extreme care during processing to protect from loss or partial degradation. Latent prints should be photographed before lifting in case they are destroyed during the lifting process.

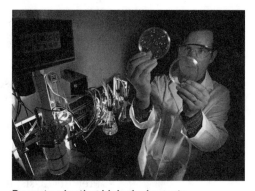

Decontaminating biological agents

The collection and packaging of all evidence is best observed by at least two individuals. There are fewer challenges to the integrity of the evidence in court if the collection and sealing process is done as soon as possible. The evidence is placed in a secure container that can be sealed with evidence tampering–proof tape. Biological materials must be placed in paper containers so that moisture can escape. The evidence packaging is sealed, dated, initialed, and labeled. The label must show a unique case item number that cannot be confused with any other item of evidence.

Chain of Custody, Evidence Sealing, and Storage

The chain of custody, the sealing of evidence, and the storage of evidence are critical to criminal proceedings. Chain of custody provides a seamless record of evidence handling and storage. The chain of custody can be described using persons and places. A law enforcement agency will designate individuals with the authority to possess or transport evidence. These individuals are trained in the proper methods for maintaining a chain of custody for items of evidence. Personnel who are not authorized to handle or store evidence must not perform these tasks. Storage locations are designated as authorized places to store evidence. Access to these locations is limited to authorized evidence custodians.

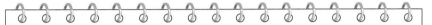

Chain of custody documents the transfer of evidence between authorized persons or between persons and places. The record of this transaction can be made in a logbook or electronic bar code system. The chain of custody transaction must include the person or place, a unique case number, date, and time if more than one transfer occurred in one day. Most important, chain of custody documentation must be made at the same time as the transaction. It cannot be made at the end of the day or the next day.

Evidence seals are sometimes the most difficult concept to describe or explain to new personnel. An evidence seal must not allow any contamination to enter the evidence container. It must not allow any evidence to leave the container. It must be destroyed when the container is opened. The evidence seal must be dated and initialed by the personnel when the seal is made.

Conversely, when an evidence container is opened, the person opening the container must document when and how the package was opened, verify the inventory of the evidence, and then reseal when analyses are completed. Any discrepancies that result in the loss, degradation, or contamination of evidence must be documented and supervisors must be notified. Noncompliance with evidence handling policy will negate any subsequent analysis. Because of the strict controls that are necessary, most agencies establish a categorical list of authorized persons and places designated for evidence handling and storage.

Conducting the Final Survey and Releasing the Scene

A final survey is done before the scene is released. This ensures that all tasks are complete. All crime scene personnel are involved in the final survey discussion to determine that tasks have been completed and documented. Documentation is reviewed for completeness and accuracy. The complete inventory of all evidence is reviewed and confirmed before its removal from the crime scene. Team members must account for all crime scene equipment and disposable supplies. Certain chemicals and body fluids, such as blood, can cause health risks for future occupants of the space. Health professionals are consulted to review any remaining health risks, as needed. The narrative for the crime scene should document that all of the steps have been completed. The narrative will include details of the crime scene release and include time of release, to whom released, by whom released, and an inventory of items secured in the search, in compliance with any court orders. Forensic experts may be needed to review the scene before its release. These individuals might include blood spatter experts, medical examiners, ballistics experts, and the prosecutor. Reentry to the scene may require an additional search warrant.

Frequently Asked Questions

Q: *What is the most difficult part of processing a crime scene?*

A: Many parts of crime scene processing are difficult. Crime scene personnel are human. The ability to remain unbiased as details of a violent crime emerge is a challenge for crime scene personnel. The most difficult situations involve children that were injured or abused, or even killed.

Q: *Is a court order needed to search a crime scene?*

A: Not always. The homeowner or legal owner of the property could grant access to the property. However, it is prudent to take the extra steps to obtain a search order when processing all crime scenes.

Q: *What is the most important step of the crime scene processing?*

A: One of the most important steps is the documentation of all the tasks performed at the scene. Tasks that are not documented will be difficult to enter into criminal trial proceedings. Direct testimony from the person who performed the task can confirm that tasks were done. However, the lack of documentation ultimately lessens the validity that the task was, in fact, performed.

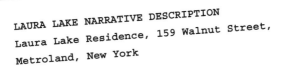

LAURA LAKE NARRATIVE DESCRIPTION
Laura Lake Residence, 159 Walnut Street,
Metroland, New York

Crime scene technician John Goodspeed has been working crime scenes for 15 years. John has seen every type of scene imaginable. He is always amazed to discover that every crime scene is a puzzle that has a solution. All that is needed is the technology, experience, and hard work that confirms or excludes a hypothesis that will solve the case.

John is a little irritated that Mary Marcel compromised the crime scene by walking in the blood spatter. Mary thought the victim was still alive when she arrived at the scene, so she ran directly to the victim to administer CPR. John realizes that treatment of the wounded is a priority, but as a result he was unable to recover any usable footprints in the blood on the floor.

The Laura Lake homicide seems routine. The victim was bludgeoned on the head with a blunt instrument that caused a great deal of blood spatter. The victim's contract landscaper, Sam Livingston, may be a suspect, but he has an alibi that cannot be confirmed at this time. He was seen working at the house for several days prior to the murder. Laura told her neighbor, Betty Smith, that she had felt sorry for him and hired him against her better judgment.

(continued)

(continued)

CRIME SCENE

Metroland Police Department
Crime Scene Narrative Description
Form CSU #3
Rev 020207

Case Number: A492	Precinct: 22	Date: April 1, 2010	First Responder: Barry Lasker	Fire Personnel:
EMT Personnel: Mary Marcel	Medical Examiner: Dr. Ali Kumar	District Attorney: Assistant District Attorney Robert Brown	Lead Detective: Detective Lieutenant Daniel Escobar	Crime Scene Team Leader: Olivia Johns
Time Start: 1100 hours	Time End: 2300 hours	Street: 159 Walnut Street	City: Metroland	County: Metro
Residence: Laura Lake Residence	Vehicle	Autopsy	Note Taker: None	Assistant: None

Received radio call at 1030 hrs while on routine patrol in Glendale neighborhood located in Precinct 22. Arrived at 159 Walnut Street, Laura Lake residence, at 1100 hours and found EMT Mary Marcel's vehicle (registration # Metro EMT #1209-112) parked in the driveway. Neighbor, Betty Smith (DOB 02/09/40), residing at 162 Walnut Street, stated loud screams came from second floor of Lake residence at about 1045 hrs. No suspect or other suspicious persons were observed after the screams were heard. However, a local handyman, Sam Livingston, had been working at the residence earlier in the week. Crime scene tape was affixed 10 feet from all sides of the residence, with an attendance log established at 1130 hrs. EMT Mary Marcel was found in the victim's upstairs bedroom, administering CPR and electronic defibrillator with negative results.

CHAPTER 5

Specific Methods of Evidence Collection, Preservation, and Documentation

Photography

Extensive use of photographs of the crime scene permits one to present, in pictorial form, all the visible physical evidence of a case. Photography aids in recording the presence of valuable evidence and permits consideration of certain types of evidence that cannot easily be brought into court. A photographic record also reveals physical evidence in place before collection, and can be referenced later in court.

Photographs include the probable path taken by the suspect to the scene, the point of entry, the exit, and the escape route. Detailed photographs are taken to show items of physical evidence prior to their removal and in the condition that they were found by the detective, first responder, or crime scene team. A crime scene photographer must be able to testify in court that the photograph accurately depicts the area shown.

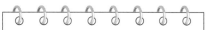

A picture is worth a thousand words. This is also true in crime scene investigation. No matter how well a detective can describe a crime scene, a photograph tells the same story even better.

An accurate photograph includes proper color, scale, and perspective. Situations in which the evidence is undergoing a state of change need to be photographed immediately. Examples are melting snow or a victim's bruises that are starting to heal. It is helpful to overlap photographs of an interior room to assist in evaluating the photographs later.

An important element in police photography is maintaining perspective. Proper photographic perspective produces the same impression of the relative position and size of visible objects as the actual objects when viewed from a particular point. Any significant distortion in the photograph will reduce, or destroy altogether, its evidentiary value.

New technology is used by many police agencies, including digital photography and videography. High resolution cameras make it possible to electronically transmit photographs taken at the scene to supervisors and other experts for evaluation. Precautions should be put in place to ensure the integrity of the digital files archived. They will be referred to as the original photographs throughout the criminal proceedings.

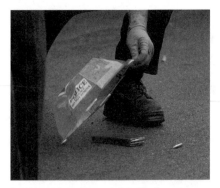

Evidence is collected, labelled, and photographed before going to the lab.

All items of evidence are photographed with an evidence tag and scale before they are moved. Photography is coordinated with the sketch preparer, the evidence recorder, and the rest of the team. The photo should include a reference point in the room or location. This will be used for correlation later in a diagram of the scene that includes all items of evidence. At a later point, the scene may need to be totally reconstructed with all items of evidence in their original locations.

All latent prints and other impression evidence are photographed before they are lifted and cast. For example, a latent print may be destroyed after it is dusted or chemically fumed. The photograph will then be identified as the latent print for comparison. Tool marks from a pry bar or any impression from a shoe may be destroyed when subjected to casting materials. If the impression evidence is destroyed in the act of collection, then the photograph acts as the original image for comparison to tools or footwear. Any blueprints, maps, or previous photographs that may assist are copied for use by all investigative personnel.

Crime scene equipment or personnel should not be shown in photographs. Evidence or other things relevant to the crime should be the only items in the photograph. Photographs must *not* be overly graphic. For example, overly graphic details of injuries may prejudice the jury or allow a perception of prejudice to surface. The photographer does not need to be qualified as an expert, but must be able to testify as to the origin of the photographs.

At a minimum, all photographs must contain the following documentation affixed to the back of the photograph:

- The direction the camera was facing
- Location of the camera
- Kind of camera
- Date and time when photograph was taken
- Who took photograph
- Shutter speed
- Lens opening
- Type of film
- Lighting
- Description of the photograph

Crime Scene Sketch

The sketch supplements the photographs. Neither photographs nor sketches stand alone to describe the scene. When done properly, both methods complement each other and clarify the crime scene for the prosecutor or jury. Crime scene sketching serves many important purposes, such as the following:

- Provides an accurate measurement of distance and sizes of items of evidence
- Identifies all items of evidence and significant objects
- Provides a reference to refresh the memory of the crime scene team
- Provides a useful tool when questioning witnesses and suspects
- Provides a permanent record of conditions not easily recorded in any other way
- Shows distances in large outdoor areas, terrain conditions, elevation, vegetation, and overall physical conditions
- Depicts the movement involved in the commission of a crime, such as the path of entry or flight, and the location of weapons

- Provides a relative scale ratio between the size of the object depicted or the distance recorded and the measurements reproduced on the sketch

The longest distance that will be shown on the final drawing should be estimated, in order to choose an appropriate scale for the sketch. A scale should be used that will provide a full reproduction of the scene on the size of paper or poster board to be used in court. The scale should optimize the size of the articles to be shown on the sketch.

The photographs and sketch provide the best way to archive all conditions at the scene before it is released. Software programs and digital cameras can provide valuable assistance in developing photographs and sketches. Large plotters and printers provide posters for display in the courtroom. Software programs can be used to enhance photographs for more clarity, such as in latent fingerprints and footwear impressions.

However, there is no substitute for how the photograph and sketch function to archive the scene. No amount of technology supplants the skills of an experienced forensic photographer and sketch developer. Some agencies have resources to provide professional artists and photographers for crime scene processing. These professionals are not essential to process all crime scenes, but can lend valuable assistance in special circumstances.

Crime Scene Search

Searching a crime scene is a tedious and demanding process. Where do you start and where do you end? No item of evidence can be missed, big or small. There may be trace evidence invisible to the naked eye, such as the DNA in saliva, blood, hair roots, semen stains, or contact surfaces. The crime scene could be any area. Most commonly, it is a room in a residence, a motor vehicle, a boat, or the open area in a yard or a field. All scenes are searched in a systematic manner with extreme thoroughness and accuracy, using a pattern or multiple patterns. There may be only one opportunity to search the scene. A search can be challenging, particularly in confined areas and in times of inclement weather and recovery of decomposed bodies.

A successful and thorough search requires preparation. The district attorney must be consulted to assess the need for a search warrant, which, in most instances, is needed. Hazards or risks need to be eliminated before the search begins. For example, there may be electrical hazards in a demolished building or biohazards from the victim's injuries and body decomposition. Chemical hazards from clandestine laboratories create very hazardous environments for crime scene personnel. Weather and the time of day are also major factors. Conditions such as brutal cold, wind, rain, or darkness may warrant postponing the search. Daylight and better weather conditions will aid the search. If a delay is necessary, measures must be taken to protect the scene.

The number of personnel deployed to the scene is limited to only those who are essential, in order to limit the possibility of contamination. Larger teams complete the job sooner but require more supervision and coordination. At a minimum, fingerprint and DNA elimination samples from all crime scene personnel may be needed to identify the sources of contamination. Elimination samples add to the analysis of the evidence and negatively affect laboratory productivity. Efforts to reduce contamination increase overall laboratory efficiency. All searchers are briefed on the scope of the search and the probative items that are important to the case. The crime scene photographer and sketch preparer are placed on standby for all found items of evidence.

Methods of Searching—Both Inside and Outside

Depending on the area to be searched, various methods can be used to search for and recover evidence systematically. These search methods include strip, grid, circle, and zone.

Strip Method

In the strip method, the area is divided into four- to eight-foot sections, depending on which is easier, and a practical outer limit of the search area is established. The searcher walks or lowers to his knees and proceeds in a straight line from end to end of the search area. The searcher then reverses direction and returns on the same path. This is repeated until the total area is searched.

Grid Method

The grid method is the same as the strip method; however when the strip method is finished, the searcher performs another strip method search *perpendicular* to the strip search pattern.

Circle Method

The circle method establishes a center point to start the search. Concentric circles or search patterns are established, beginning at the center point and working out to the outer perimeter of the search area. This method may be of value if there is a certain area that is more significant than other areas of the search. Investigators can focus resources on the area that has the most potential for probative items of evidence at the very beginning of the investigation.

A 360-degree perspective is maintained throughout the search. There may be evidence in trees, bushes, on rooftops, or ceilings. Searchers should not forget to look up!

Zone Method

The zone method establishes quadrants of search areas that are systematically searched until all areas are completed. This type of search is most useful when searching a very large area in an outside environment.

Searching Indoors

Two crime scene members search a room as a team. One member observes the floor and lower portion of the wall and the other observes the upper portion of the wall and the ceiling. Next, the crime scene members reverse the assignments, repeating the search of the room. All items in the room are searched after the floor, walls, and ceilings.

Hard surface floors receive special attention. Blood spatter and footprints are recoverable from these surfaces. A variety of lighting techniques and chemical enhancements can reveal trace and impression evidence on these surfaces. If it is not practical to recover this type of evidence early in the investigation, these areas are protected with butcher paper or other suitable material. The most practical method to detect evidence on these types of floors is the use of oblique lighting with normal high intensity flashlights or alternate wavelength light sources. All items of evidence found are placed on the sketch, photographed, packaged, sealed, and added to the total evidence inventory. Chemical agents that are sensitive to blood are also used to expose blood spatter and smears that are invisible under normal conditions.

Searching a Vehicle

A vehicle is systematically searched in the same manner as a room or residence, keeping in mind the overall scope of the search. If the crime scene

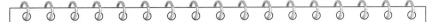

Outside surfaces of windows can provide valuable evidence. Suspects often peer inside a residence before breaking in. In the process, they may place a hand or forehead against the window glass. This contact can leave a fingerprint or trace of DNA.

team is looking to place an individual within the interior of the vehicle, then the seats, floor, dashboard, and ceiling are divided into quadrants or zones. There may be circumstances when the seat cover requires microscopic analysis at the laboratory. Seat covers are removed and packaged, protecting all surfaces from contamination and loss of trace evidence. Hit-and-run accidents present a specific set of trace evidence considerations. The task of the crime scene personnel is to find traces of the vehicle upon the clothing or body of the victim and traces of the victim's clothing or body on the vehicle. Trace particles of plastic, paint, and glass from the vehicle are often found on the victim. Trace amounts of hair, blood, or the victim's clothing are often found on the grill or undercarriage of the vehicle.

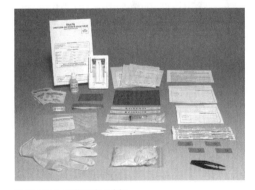

Evidence collection kit

The search of a crime scene is the fundamental beginning of the forensic process. The crime scene team will only have one chance to recognize, collect, and protect the evidence. They will probably never return to the scene after it is released to the legal owners. The challenge for the crime scene team is to use the Locard principle and find the "trace evidence left from every contact."

THE CRIME SCENE: HOW FORENSIC SCIENCE WORKS

Frequently Asked Questions

Q: *What is the average time to search a scene?*

A: The time varies with the type of crime. A burglary scene may be processed within a few hours. A homicide team may take several days or even weeks. The crime scene team is concerned with being thorough and not missing one item of evidence. They should not be pressured. They are done when they are done.

Q: *Are there any specialty programs that teach crime scene processing?*

A: Most programs are taught within police departments. Several colleges have developed crime scene processing programs with specific courses at the undergraduate and graduate level.

Q: *What is the future of crime scene processing?*

A: New detection technologies for biological materials (DNA) will revolutionize crime scene processing. Miniaturized chips will perform DNA analyses that will compare unknown DNA profiles to databases of known suspects. This will all happen at the crime scene. Lower detection limits and power of discrimination will increase the demand for these new technologies.

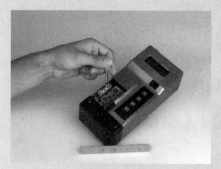

Handheld device/portable lab

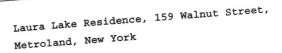

Laura Lake Residence, 159 Walnut Street, Metroland, New York

CRIME SCENE

Quality Assurance Supervisor Carol Lent reviews all documentation from major crimes submitted to Metroland County Forensic Laboratory. Her job is to prepare and monitor all processes to ensure accreditation is maintained with the American Society of Crime Laboratory Directors/Laboratory Accreditation Board International ISO/IEC 17025:2005 program. Scientists document what they do contemporaneously with the performance of the task. For example, photographs at the scene are initialed and dated to indicate who took the photographs and when they were taken. The laboratory director has also assigned Carol to provide an "ISO overview" for all homicide cases. The director realizes that her years of experience in serology analysis and crime scene processing are valuable intangible assets.

Carol misses the challenge of solving crimes at the scene, but she does not miss the late hours and being "on call" 24/7. Homicides never seem to occur during normal work hours: 8 A.M. to 5 P.M., Monday through Friday. Carol has strong fundamental knowledge of microbiology but lacks hands-on skills needed to operate DNA technologies. The new equipment requires full-time operators with specific computer expertise and daily casework responsibilities. Carol envies the "new kids on the block" and feels that the job has passed her by.

While checking photographs for initials and dates, Carol recognizes that one photograph depicts an unknown blockade that caused an absence of blood spatter on the floor next to the victim. Blockades interrupt the trajectory of airborne blood spatter. If the blockade is later removed then there is a conspicuous absence of blood spatter in that location. The legs of the suspect, chairs, lamps, plant stands, and many other objects cause blockage of the blood spatter

(continued)

(continued)

during the crime. Carol wonders if any items that might have caused the blockade were submitted for examination of the blood spatter.

Metroland Police Department
Photograph Record
CSU Document #2
Revised 043010

Date: April 1, 2010	Precinct and Case #: A492	Photographer Name: Kathy Fieger Photographer Badge #132	Start Time: 1300 hours	End Time: 2300 hours
Supervisor Investigator: Detective Lieutenant Daniel Escobar	Crime Scene Team Leader: Olivia Johns	Weather: Clear	Camera Type: Canon MSC3000	Film Type or Digital Media: Digital—10Mpixel
Street Address: 159 Walnut Street	City: Metroland	County: Metro County	State: New York	Camera Filters: None
Complainant: Betty Smith	Defendant: Unknown	Deceased: Laura Lake	DOB: 06/04/45	Injuries: Multiple blunt trauma
	Residence: Yes	Vehicle	Autopsy	Scale Used: Fischer Scientific Multi-gradient

Photo #1	Exterior front elevation
Photo #2	Exterior right side elevation
Photo #3	Exterior left side elevation
Photo #4	Exterior rear side elevation

(continued)

CRIME SCENE

Photo #5	Aerial 3,000 feet
Photo #6	Aerial 6,000 feet
Photo #7	Ceiling bedroom
Photo #8	Floor bedroom
Photo #9	Outside wall bedroom
Photo #10	South wall bedroom
Photo #11	East wall bedroom
Photo #12	West wall bedroom
Photo #13	Blood spatter on floor near victim—5 feet distance
Photo #14	Blood spatter on floor near victim—2 feet distance
Photo #15	Blood spatter on floor near victim—1 foot distance
Photo #16	
Photo #17	
Photo #18	
Photo #19	
Photo #20	
Photo #21	
Photo #22	
Photo #23	
Photo #24	
Photo #25	

CHAPTER 6

Latent Fingerprints and Blood

Latent Prints

Fingerprints are one of the most important types of evidence collected at the crime scene. DNA has stolen the media spotlight in recent years, but fingerprints have stood the test of time as evidence that the suspect was at the crime scene. Fingerprints are limited only in the sense that they cannot provide the *time* when the suspect was at the scene.

The science of fingerprint identification uses the distinctive ridges found on the tips of our fingers. Known fingerprints (Ks) are collected from suspects at the time of arrest and are called "10 prints" as they provide fingerprints for all 10 fingers. Questioned fingerprints (Qs) are the latent fingerprints found at crime scenes and on items of evidence.

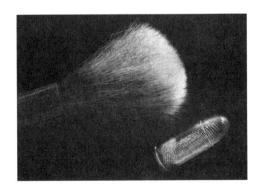

Dusting for latent prints

Fingerprints are formed from material on the fingers, such as grease or blood, that is pressed upon a surface. Prints are also formed from natural oils secreted by the fingers. Every circumstance imaginable can lead to the formation of fingerprints on an evidence item. Smooth, nonporous surfaces like glass and plastic are ideal places to find

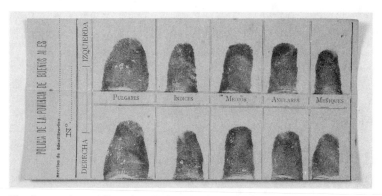

The fingerprints of Francisco Rojas, the first person convicted of
murder through fingerprint evidence

fingerprints. Irregular, rough, or soft surfaces, such as clothing or rugs, are
generally not conducive to forming good prints.

A variety of techniques use powders and chemicals to develop
latent fingerprints. A lift, or lifted fingerprint, is formed when a piece
of adhesive tape is placed over a developed latent print and pulled
away. The latent print adheres to the tape and then the tape is placed
upon a glossy white or black "latent lift backer" card. The backer is
then labeled properly and retained as evidence. Extensive photography
is used during the development and lifting process because the print
can be destroyed by any of the development or collection techniques.

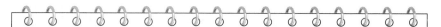

Police supervisors, crime scene personnel, and first responders learn very
quickly how *not* to contaminate a crime scene. In other words, Stay Out!
Only those who need to go in are allowed in. There is no "ego" access.

DNA or fingerprints from police personnel can contaminate the scene.
If this contamination takes place, their profiles will be collected by crime
scene technicians, resulting in latent prints and DNA profiles developed at
the lab. Crime scene personnel and police supervisors do not want to learn
in an official lab report presented in court that their DNA or fingerprints
were found at the scene due to contamination.

If the latent lift is destroyed, then the photograph is used to replace
it for identification purposes. As with all trace evidence, elimination
prints—or "eliminators"—must be obtained from all individuals who

have had legal access to the property in question. This includes crime scene and first responder personnel.

Fingerprints and DNA are the two main forensic disciplines that can prove the identity of an individual who has been at a crime scene or in contact with an item of evidence. To date, no two individuals have been found to have the same fingerprints. Only identical twins have the same DNA profile.

It is possible to find a latent print in the blood of the victim. This is a double winner or home run. This is because DNA from the blood (Q) is the medium for the formation of the latent fingerprint (Q) which can be compared with the 10 print fingerprint card of the suspect (K) and the control blood from the victim (K). Other evidence would be insignificant and may not even need to be analyzed in this situation. The resulting matches in these two types of evidence, although rare, may result in the closure of the case at the highest criminal charge.

Developing Latent Prints

The crime scene technician is aware of the many contact or "touch" surfaces that are possible sources of latent fingerprints and traces of DNA. Chemicals and powders can be used to develop latent fingerprints on these surfaces, as they may not be visible in natural light. Some of these materials are hazardous and must be handled and used with proper protective equipment. The Material Safety Data Sheet (MSDS) for all chemicals must be consulted for appropriate precautions.

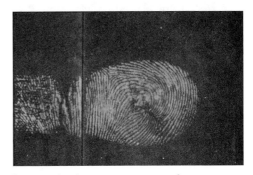

Latent print from non-porous surface

For example, aerosols from fine particulates in latent print powders can be hazardous. The following techniques are available to crime scene technicians and latent print examiners:

- Ninhydrin
- Silver nitrate
- Physical developer
- Iodine fuming
- Luminescence

- Amido black
- Gentian violet
- Ardrox
- Rhodamine G
- Cyanoacrylate ester fuming (superglue)

The lifting of a latent print is a very delicate process. Perfect latent fingerprints can be successfully lifted from a variety of surfaces. If the surface appears to be difficult, the technician may choose to remove the surface (door frame, window) and submit it to the laboratory to prepare for lifting in a controlled environment. The technician will prepare detailed notes, sketches, and photographs before attempting any type of lift. The technician will choose a latent lift backer color that will contrast with the color of the latent lift (black on white). A mark is placed on the surface of the item next to but not on the latent print. The object upon which the latent print was developed must also be treated as evidence and preserved. The latent lift on the adhesive is then carefully placed upon the lift backer. The appropriate evidence identification information is written on the back of the latent print backer card. Figure 6.1 provides an example of a method for latent fingerprint development.

Blood Stains and Blood Spatter Patterns

DNA technology has revolutionized forensic science. The power of DNA technology complements latent fingerprint analyses and allows identification of many more suspects at crime scenes. There are times when a crime scene technician becomes overwhelmed by the amount of blood at a scene. The collection of blood must be planned carefully to submit the most probative items to the laboratory for analysis. Laboratories do not have the capacity to analyze all blood-related items present at the scene.

Blood can be categorized as wet blood, dry blood, and spatter blood. Spatter blood can be both wet and dry, and is used for reconstructing the crime scene. Blood spatter investigative techniques will assist the crime scene technician in selecting probative items of blood for analyses. A particularly violent crime

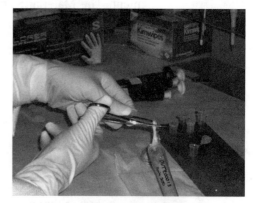

Forensic scientist cutting swab from blood soaked garment

FIGURE 6.1 *Example of a Method for Latent Print Development*

Abstract Latent Fingerprint Method Manual
Method # 11
Revision 123
Effective 2.2.07

Ninhydrin Method for Blood Print Enhancement

SCOPE: Ninhydrin is sensitive to the proteins in blood. Ninhydrin is best used on porous surfaces such as paper. This chemical causes the latent fingerprint to produce a violet-blue color.

SAFETY CONSIDERATIONS: Review the MSDS literature for ethyl acetate, methanol, ninhydrin, and freon TF. All of these chemicals are extremely dangerous. Use the proper personal protective equipment.

REAGENTS:
- Ninhydrin
- Methanol
- Ethyl acetate
- Freon TF

PREPARATION: Measure the appropriate amount of reagents in a beaker that is placed in a container of warm water. Slowly mix until all reagents are completely dissolved.

CONTROLS AND STANDARDS: Place your own fingerprints on a suitable control (paper) as a positive standard. Cut into strips and place in the ninhydrin solution. Also, place in the solution the strips of the same paper with no latent prints and designate as a blank standard. Place the strips in the proper environment of heat and humidity. If your own prints develop on the positive standard and there is no reaction on the blank, then proceed with the questioned evidence. Document the result of the standard test in the reagent log.

PROCEDURE: All work is done in a fume hood. In a tray large enough to contain the evidence add enough solution to cover the evidence. Completely cover all of the evidence with the solution. Use a tong or forceps to handle the evidence. Remove and properly dry the items.

INTERPRETATION OF RESULTS: The prints developed by the ninhydrin may only last for days, or may last for years. The prints may also keep developing and become less distinct over time. Be prepared to photograph all stages of development to gain the best possible representation of the latent fingerprint.

Adapted from U.S. Department of Justice, *Chemical Formulas and Processing Guide for the Development of Latent Fingerprints,* 1994.

CAUTION: THIS IS AN ABSTRACT OF A METHOD AND NOT INTENDED FOR ANY USE OR APPLICATION will generate a large amount of blood spatter and the crime scene team should collect as much as possible. Several hundred wet and dry stains are probable. The notes, sketch, and photography of blood evidence before it is collected is critical.

Crime scene technicians should not attempt to remove blood from an item. Rather, the item should be collected, protected, and submitted to the laboratory. The stain may be rendered useless for analysis unless it is removed correctly. When possible, the item bearing the stain is submitted in its entirety along with fluid samples of blood control standards from the victim (K), deceased, defendant, suspect, and any others involved.

Precautions must be in place to prevent contamination and bacterial degradation of blood evidence. It is best for team members to use all disposable tools one time only in the collection process. Then they are disposed of in biohazard containers according to the Occupational Safety and Health Administration's Bloodborne Pathogens Standard. This includes forceps, scalpels, and gloves. The crime scene technician must change gloves after touching each item.

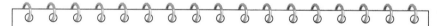

Technicians must be protected from blood born pathogens and noxious odors present at the crime scene. Personal protective equipment such as masks, gloves, and Tyvek clothing prevent exposure to pathogens and odors. Conversely, foreign material from crime scene personnel must not contaminate the evidence. Top priority is always the safety of the crime scene personnel.

The crime scene team must remember to *touch it once and do it right*. When in doubt, the team can call the laboratory for advice or assistance.

Wet bloodstains can be collected from nonabsorbent surfaces with a sterilized, saline solution prepared by the laboratory. A disposable sterilized swab or eyedropper can be used to collect a sample of the bloodstain. The blood sample is then placed in a blood tube recommended by the laboratory. Absorbent materials such as clothing, rugs, or bedding will require submission to the laboratory. All items must be dried as much as possible before submission to the laboratory. A sample of the material without any blood must also be submitted as the blank control. Irregular and absorbent materials, such as wood, can be soaked with a large amount of blood. Some of the stain can be diluted with sterilized water from the laboratory or a dry sterilized swab can be used to collect the mixture. Dried bloodstains are some of the best samples collected at a crime scene.

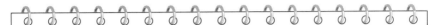

The Biotracks program in New York City and other major metropolitan police departments has successfully solved many lesser offenses, such as burglary and property crimes. The Biotracks program targets the collection of biological evidence from lesser offense crime scenes. Many of these lesser cases are linked to other property crimes and even violent crimes such as sexual assaults and homicides. Burglars often injure themselves, leaving drops of blood upon entering the residence. Dried blood is one of the most effective types of evidence collected that result in DNA profiles. These "biotracks" are the Locard items of the 21st century.

Blood spatter analysis is one of the most effective tools used in crime scene reconstruction and must be considered when processing the scene. A technician trained in blood spatter views the crime scene from a very different perspective. Dr. Paul Kirk used the technique in the early 1950s at the Marilyn Sheppard crime scene in Cleveland, Ohio. This homicide case is documented in Bernard F. Conner's book, *Tailspin.*

Analyzing the trajectory of the spatter can identify the source location of the spattered blood. For example, the angle of trajectory and direction of flight of the blood spatter can be inferred from its shape. A perfectly round drop of blood is the result of a vertical drop to a perpendicular flat surface. A very long, oblong shape documents the direction of flight and angle of impact.

There is a difference between high-speed impact and low-speed impact blood spatter. Ballistic wounds create high-speed blood spatter consistent with smaller particles or mistlike patterns. Low-speed spatter will result in larger drops of blood.

Blockades create areas in which there is no blood spatter. These are very significant. A suspect, witness, or victim can block the spatter of blood with their body during the commission of the crime. This causes a distinct area on the floor or wall with no blood spatter due to the blockade created by the victim's or suspect's legs or body. Bodies or furniture may have been

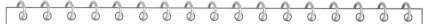

In the late 1980s, a homicide investigation in a small village in upstate New York involved a girl who was severely beaten on the head with a baseball bat in a poolroom. The floor, pool table, and ceiling were covered with blood spatter that emanated from the location of the victim's head. There were two blockades resulting from the legs of the suspect.

The key to solving this crime was to find the suspect and obtain his pants in order to find the blood spatter blockaded at the scene. The suspect was found the same day as the crime. Preliminary tests showed blood on his pants. The suspect claimed the blood resulted from a bloody nose during a fight in the bar, and not from the victim. Close examination of his pants, however, revealed that the entire blood spatter consisted of horizontal spatter at a low angle, not vertical drops of blood. When presented with the blood spatter evidence, the suspect admitted to the crime.

Blood spatter analysis is common sense *plus* specialized training. Evidence from the scene that *does not correlate* with suspect/witness statements solves crimes.

moved before the crime scene team arrived at the scene. Blood spatter can help show how the scene was compromised. Blood spatter analysis can be used effectively during interviews with suspects.

Many diverse biological materials are commonly collected for DNA analyses. These include the following:

- Blood, liquid
- Hair (with roots)
- Blood, wet/dry stains
- Body tissue/organs
- Semen, liquid
- Dental pulp
- Semen, wet/dry stains
- Bone marrow
- Saliva
- Fetal material (for criminal parentage analysis)
- Skin residue (i.e., on eyeglasses or hatbands)
- Fecal material

Fingerprints and blood are significant items that need to be recognized, collected, and preserved at a crime scene. Circumstances where blood and fingerprints are combined to form one item of evidence result in a bloody fingerprint. How do personnel collect and analyze these types of evidence without compromising any individual value of the items? In short: very carefully and as a team. The crime scene team will contact the laboratory and ask for assistance in this type of evidence collection and analyses. The bloody fingerprint may even be cut out of a floor or wall and transported to the labo-

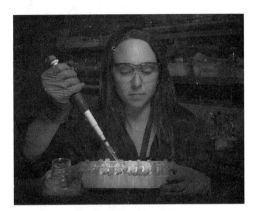

Scientist pipetting biological fluids

ratory. The crime scene team, latent print examiner, and DNA scientist will work together within a controlled laboratory environment to maximize the value of the evidence. The DNA scientist will often remove a small or microscopic particle of blood for analysis from a nonprobative area of the latent fingerprint. Extensive photography by the crime scene team is performed during all steps of this process.

Frequently Asked Questions

Q: *What types of latent fingerprint development materials affect DNA analyses?*

A: The crime scene technician will always check with the scientists at the laboratory before applying latent fingerprint reagents that may affect DNA analyses. The following latent print techniques or reagents may affect DNA analyses:

- UV radiation
- Physical developer
- Magnetic powder
- Multimetal deposition (MMD)

The following latent print reagents do not affect DNA analyses:

- Black powder
- Aluminum powder
- Ninhydrin
- DAB
- Cyanoacrylate glue fuming
- Sticky-side powder
- Luminol
- DFO
- Amido black
- Strong white light
- White powder

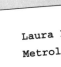

Laura Lake Residence, 159 Walnut Street, Metroland, New York

CRIME SCENE

Latent print examiner, Larry Poler, completed his two-year training as a latent fingerprint examiner last year. Larry is now able to work unsupervised on major cases, such as the Laura Lake homicide. His supervisor is from the old school, and believes there are always latent fingerprints left at the scene by the suspect. You just have to find them. Larry has now processed for latent prints over 100 items of evidence that were sent to the laboratory. The only prints he has recovered and identified belonged to the victim, EMT Mary Marcel, and other first responders. Larry also went to the scene to process any stationary or fixed items or surfaces for possible latent prints. Similarly, the only fingerprints he found matched individuals with legal access to the residence.

The investigators have not been able to eliminate Sam Livingston as a suspect for this crime. The collection and identification of suspect Sam Livingston's fingerprints at the crime scene would place him at the scene but would not indicate *when* he was at the scene. Investigators know Sam had a contract with the victim to do landscaping. If any of Sam's prints are found inside the residence, however, Sam would have to explain his reason for being inside the home.

Larry spent one full week at the crime scene and four full weeks, including weekends, at the laboratory to process fingerprint evidence and comparisons for Ks and Qs. During this time, he left the lab only one afternoon to attend his young daughter's birthday party. After five weeks of work, Larry's report only states the identification of latent fingerprints from known individuals having legal access to the residence, or "eliminators." Larry and his boss are disappointed, but realize that not all cases have a "smoking gun," or probative latent fingerprints that match a suspect.

CHAPTER 7

Collection and Protection of Questioned Documents, Fibers, and Firearms

Questioned Documents

One of the most extensive apprenticeships in the forensic sciences is that of the questioned documents (QD) examiner. Currently, there are no undergraduate or graduate academic programs that provide specialized training in this area. The key to acquiring expertise in this discipline is to work with an experienced QD examiner in a lab that handles a large variety of QD casework. Training typically takes three to five years under the tutelage of a professional mentor.

Large forensic science lab systems maintain at least two document examiners in order to provide peer review of each other's work. Geographical areas that have a small number of QD cases typically cannot justify the expense of hiring a QD examiner. These labs send their QD cases to state or federal laboratories for analysis.

Questioned document analysis typically provides support for investigative opinions. Rarely does QD provide a categorical opinion that will include or exclude a questioned document (Q) when compared to control documents (Ks).

What are the known (K) and questioned (Q) items for QD examiners? QD involves three categories of analysis: tools, surfaces, and handwriting. The first analysis is the tool used to make the mark. A tool could be any type of printer, typewriter, pen, or pencil. The second analysis is the actual surface imprinted upon by the writing tool. This could include paper of any kind, as well as other types of surfaces. The third analysis is handwriting. A known exemplar of handwriting is compared to the questioned document. Thus, QD examines writing tools and surfaces, comparing the handwriting in question to known samples of the suspect's handwriting.

Most document examinations analyze printing or writing on paper. The crime scene team must remember that saliva from adhesive envelope flaps may contain DNA. The crime scene team and first responder must take pre-cautions to avoid contaminating the document with their own DNA. Basic handling procedures are essential, including using disposable forceps and changing gloves between collections of items of evidence. The document must be preserved in the same condition that it was found, with no bending or folding. Charred documents are best collected by sliding a paper under the document and placing it within a protective box.

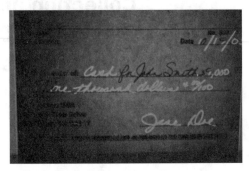

Forged check

The original document must be submitted to the laboratory for analysis and comparison. Photographs are of no value for examining erasures, obliterations, chemical reagents, sidelight-ing, indentations, or latent fingerprint development. Photography—not a photocopier—is used to make copies of documents. Pressures exerted by the photocopier may damage the original document, indented writings, erasures, latent fingerprints, trace evidence, and obliterations. If copies of the original documents are needed by detectives, then the document is photographed extensively *before* sending to the laboratory.

Microscopic and chemical analyses may be performed on the original controls (Ks) for comparisons to the unknowns (Qs). Known writings form the bulk of controls used for QD analyses. The writings can be from diaries, notebooks, check receipts, letters, or any other document that was completed by the suspect or victim in the recent past. Control samples from victims or suspects must be obtained. A court order may be required before collecting control samples from suspects. The same writing material that was used in the questioned document is used in the control. Dictation is the preferred method of obtaining control samples. The suspect will not have prior knowledge of the requested writing and will provide a more spontaneous sample. At least 5 and preferably 10 control samples should be obtained from the suspect.

The following is a general list of controls used for document examination:

- *Paper.* Paper is protected from contamination with proper handling and packaging. A variety of paper types, weights, and manufacturers use specific production techniques that can then be compared.
- *Writing instruments.* Markers, ballpoint pens, fountain pens, and pencils are the majority of writing instruments used in handwriting or marking. Production lots of these items are quite large and it is difficult to determine unique chemical or physical properties. It may be possible to exclude a writing instrument as the source of the writing.
- *Date/time stamps and rubber stamps.* Stamps are very useful for a known control. There will be unique, even microscopic, imperfections on the stamp that may be seen on the questioned document.
- *Printers.* Ink-jet, laser jet, photocopiers, and the ink or powders associated with their use are useful for comparison to questioned documents. Physical imperfections in the faceplates and rollers of these machines may transfer to the questioned documents. Chemical analyses of the inks and powders may be unique or exclusionary.
- *Handwriting.* The majority of document cases are handwriting analyses. The team must decide what letters, groups of letters, or phrases are probative in the questioned document and ensure these phrase or letter groupings are used within the control writing. Dictation and collection of control writings previously done by the suspect are used for controls in signature or handwriting analyses.

Fibers

Natural and synthetic fibers are everywhere. Clothing, automobiles, and furnishings in homes all contain a myriad of fibers.

The crime scene team considers the many possibilities for transfer of fibers between suspects and victims. Fiber evidence is very small and fragile. Collection and protection of fiber evidence is critical. If not

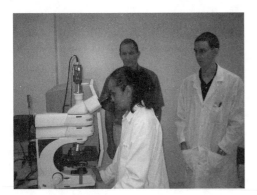

Confocal microscopy

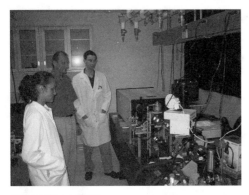

Research on fibers

done properly, fibers can be lost or contaminated. Static electricity can cause a fiber to literally jump off an item and disappear.

Examination of fibers is performed with microscopes and other analytical instruments in the lab. The crime scene team must know where to find and collect fiber evidence and transport it to the laboratory without loss. Fibers are usually found on a secondary item. The best policy is to collect and transport the secondary item in its entirety to the laboratory. Laboratory scientists are best equipped to remove and protect fibers for analysis.

As an example, fibers can transfer between the clothing of a suspect and the carpet or seats of an automobile. Properly collecting the suspect's clothing and vehicular carpets or seat coverings is necessary to allow for control and questioned fiber comparison. The laboratory scientists will collect the questioned fibers suitable for microscopic and chemical comparisons.

Forensic vacuums can also be used at crime scenes. A variety of macro and micro filters are used to sort and collect fibers from secondary objects.

The following are the major categories of fibers:

- Blends of synthetic and natural fibers (polyester and cotton)
- Animal hair (wool)
- Vegetable fibers (cotton)
- Synthetic fibers (rayon, nylon, plastics, polyester)
- Mineral fibers (glass wool)

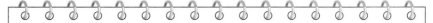

A case in Atlanta, Georgia, in the late 1970s and early 1980s brought fiber evidence into the spotlight of the forensic community. In 1982, Wayne Williams was convicted of killing two children, largely as a result of fiber and hair evidence collected from the crime scenes, victims, and Williams's residence. The police subsequently closed 22 other homicides attributed to Williams.

It is interesting that there is now mounting pressure to apply DNA technology to the Williams case. Dog hair was one of the comparisons used to convict Williams in the Atlanta murders. The defense community is now asking for DNA comparison of the dog hair and other hair, to either support or exclude microscopic comparisons originally performed on the hair evidence.

Firearms and Ammunition

Firearms are the main weapons used in homicide and serious assault cases. Detectives, first responders, and crime scene technicians must be familiar with different types of firearms. Firearms examiners in the laboratory are, for the most part, sworn police officers who have experience from patrol assignments and possess advanced skills. Some agencies include civilian personnel in the firearms unit, but this is unusual and may be restricted by police labor relation contracts.

Every firearm recovered is considered loaded and ready to fire. The safety of personnel is always the first priority when handling, transporting, and examining firearm evidence at the crime scene or the laboratory. All law enforcement agencies provide firearm safety programs for line officers. Firearm evidence consists of four main categories: firearms, ammunition, spent cartridge cases, and projectiles.

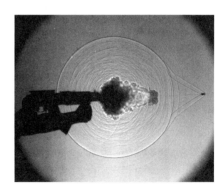

Analysis of projectile in motion

The firearms examiner performs two major tasks: operability, and microscopic comparisons of projectiles and casings. Comparisons can be made between questioned (Q) projectiles and casings found at multiple scenes (by comparing a string of multiple shootings to determine if the same weapon was used), or by comparison to test fires from a known weapon (K). The known weapon can be found at the scene or in the possession or control of the suspect.

The crime scene examiner takes detailed notes and photographs the condition of the weapon before the weapon is collected and packaged. For example, the crime scene technician notes the position of the safety, cylinder, slide, hammer, and clip, and the relationship to the projectiles and cartridges. These relationships may be critical for crime scene reconstruction, done later in the investigation. The weapon must also be unloaded or put into safe mode before packaging or transporting to the laboratory. If the crime scene technician decides the steps needed to unload the weapon will compromise trace evidence, then the firearms examiner from the laboratory must be consulted or even go to the scene. Trace evidence must be preserved and protected. There may be hairs, fibers, fingerprints, or blood on or in the firearm. Blood and clothing fibers may blow back on the weapon or inside the barrel when the weapon is close to the victim. The laboratory should be consulted when this type of probative trace evidence is present. A multidiscipline team consisting of the firearms examiner, latent print examiner, and DNA scientist will work on the item together to maximize information developed from the evidence.

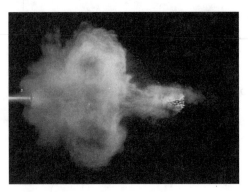

Firearm muzzle blast

The crime scene technician takes detailed notes on the location and condition of all ammunition that is taken from the weapon when it is unloaded. The exact location of ammunition in the cylinder or clip, and whether the cartridge is fired or unfired, is critical information. This could be extremely helpful in determining if the weapon was used for suicide, accidental shooting, or homicide. Weapons found underwater should be put in a container, submerged in the same water, and taken to the laboratory immediately. The rusting process accelerates if the weapon is allowed to air-dry before examination.

Firearms must be marked, tagged, packaged, and sealed the same as any other type of evidence. The crime scene technician must know how to "bag and tag" weapons without obliterating or causing the loss of trace evidence. There are weapons that can be marked directly on a nonprobative surface (under grips or frame) and there are weapons, casings, and projectiles that would be best left unmarked and placed in fully labeled containers. The crime scene technician will gain experience over time in consultation with the firearms examiners within the laboratory.

Two types of gunshot residue (GSR) can be recognized and collected by specially trained crime scene examiners. The first is formed from the high temperature and pressure developed within the chamber of a weapon immediately upon discharge. The high temperature and pressure vaporize the lead, antimony, and barium found in the primer, gunpowder, and projectile. The lead, antimony, and barium then cool and solidify into unique spherical particles that can be visualized using a scanning electron microscope. The second form of GSR is the gunpowder that was not ignited when the weapon was fired. There is always a small amount of unignited gunpowder that is expelled from the barrel of the weapon. This gunpowder can be collected from surfaces within a short radius of the fired weapon. The laboratory performs test fires with similar weapons and ammunition to establish the distribution patterns and range of both types of GSR.

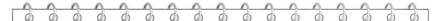

GSR came to the rescue of two troopers transporting a mentally disturbed criminal from the courtroom to a psychiatric care facility. Upon exiting the vehicle at the psychiatric facility, the criminal wrestled a trooper's gun from its holster. The two troopers and the criminal grappled for the weapon for several minutes and the weapon was expelled from the mêlée 15 feet straight up in the air. The weapon discharged as it hit the hood of the police car, striking the criminal in the leg. The criminal claimed the troopers tried to execute him in the parking lot.

Examination for GSR on the troopers' and victim's hands and clothing was negative. There was a large tool mark along with GSR found on the fender of the police car. This confirmed the location of the weapon when the discharge took place. The two troopers learned a lesson about the value of GSR, blockades, and physical evidence.

GSR vapor exits the weapon from the gaps around the cylinder, breech, slide, and barrel in a distinct pattern. The distribution pattern of the GSR can be critical in crime scene reconstruction. Has the GSR been blockaded (similar to blood spatter blockades) by objects, the victim, or suspect? GSR may be found on these blockade objects. This information can be critical to support or disprove statements from victims or suspects.

Frequently Asked Questions

Q: *Is it difficult to collect and preserve firearm evidence at the crime scene?*

A: Yes. Collecting firearm evidence is time consuming. The force and trajectory of projectiles and casings create unlimited possibilities for the location of these items. Safety is the most important criterion. A recovered firearm must be made "safe" before any processing can begin.

Q: *How do crime scene technicians become knowledgeable in the variety of weapons and ammunition encountered at the crime scene?*

A: The crime scene technician must apply for and attend all internal agency and external firearm training classes available. Training is supplemented by forming mentor relationships with experienced crime scene technicians and firearms examiners. This is a very specialized group of experts. There are no colleges or university programs that provide specialized training in firearm evidence collection or examination.

Q: *How are cartridges and gunpowder residues examined?*

A: Unspent gunpowder residue emitted from the barrel is used to determine distance between the weapon and victim. The crime scene team needs to be aware of GSR and unspent powder distribution patterns and collect the appropriate evidence for comparisons to the same weapon and ammunition.

All cartridges and projectiles must be accounted for when processing a crime scene. Multiple firings may require an exhaustive search of the neighborhood to find all cartridges and projectiles embedded in different structures, the landscape, highways, or sewer systems. Embedded projectiles must be carefully cut out without marking or deforming the projectile in any way.

CHAPTER 8

Collection of Impressions, Hair, and Toxicology Specimens

Footwear and Tires

Footwear and tires create similar imprint and impression evidence. *Imprints* are created when footwear or tires contact a hard surface. Dirt or dust is transferred to the surface, replicating the original pattern of the tire or footwear tread. Oil, paint, or another foreign substance transfers from the tire or footwear to the hard surface. *Impressions* are created when footwear or tires compress, leaving a reverse impression of the tread in a substrate, such as soil, mud, sand, or snow.

Prints from footwear and tires are commonly found at crime scenes. Crime scene personnel must carefully examine all entrances and exits to the scene, as they may have been used by the criminal. A large roll of butcher paper can be placed down in traffic areas to preserve the site and to allow collection later during crime scene processing. Footwear and tire imprints must also be protected from the environment. Cardboard boxes or other suitable material can protect imprints and impressions from the rain, snow, and traffic.

Blood is often found on the floor where a violent crime has taken place. Individuals such as first responders, emergency medical technicians, or firefighters may walk through the blood evidence when responding to the crime. These individuals must provide their footwear to the laboratory to be eliminated as the source of the footwear imprints.

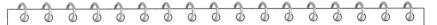

MARK'S STORY

"Invisible" bloody footprints are dramatic items of evidence. Reagents are sprayed with a fine mist over suspected areas at the crime scene. They react chemically with blood and display a blue or purple color.

We investigated one case involving an elderly couple who were murdered in their small bungalow. The flooring was a light-colored linoleum tile. One partial bloody footwear imprint could be seen near the bodies, but no other imprints were visible with the naked eye. The reagent luminol revealed footwear imprints leading from the bodies to the front door. Several of these footwear imprints were developed and photographed. The resulting prints had such striking detail that when compared to the suspect's shoes, they were found to be an exact match. Thus, "invisible footprints" led to the arrest and ultimate prosecution of the suspect.

A variety of chemical agents help visualize trace or invisible amounts of blood on nonporous tile and wood flooring. Most reagents react with the iron in blood hemoglobin and change color or fluoresce to reveal the imprint. However, iron-containing compounds and other similar chemicals will also cause a positive reaction. Crime scene technicians must also follow safety precautions and use only the amount of reagent necessary to develop the print. This is critical in that the crime scene must not be unnecessarily saturated with reagents, creating a hazard similar to a chemical spill.

Luminol is commonly used as a reagent to enhance trace invisible amounts of blood created by a footwear imprint. During this process, the footwear imprints must be photographed continuously as the chemical reaction develops, because some areas will become overly developed and less distinct. The developed footwear imprint (Q) is compared against the shoes worn by individuals who had access to the scene, including the suspect (K).

The crime scene team must protect these impressions from potential damage or contamination. Footprints and impressions can yield a categorical positive match to footwear due to macro and microscopic wear marks on the sole of the shoe. Several small nicks or unique wear marks on the footwear or tire may be enough for the experienced scientist to give the opinion that the suspect's shoe or tire (K) was the source of the imprint developed from the crime scene (Q). There may also be a transfer of material from the surface of the imprint or impression to the footwear or tire. Grease, hair, fibers, blood, or soil may transfer from the impression or imprint to the footwear or tire. The most significant transfer material is blood. DNA analyses of the blood can provide a match to the victim's blood, placing the shoes or tires at the scene of the crime. Other trace material is supportive but not as probative as DNA. Of course, all of these comparisons can exclude footwear or tires from causing the imprints or impressions. Exclusions are just as significant as positive matches.

Footwear and tire castings are made from plaster or dental stone. Crime scene technicians thoroughly practice these techniques in a variety of conditions before attempting this task at a crime scene. An excellent casting can be ruined if not done properly. Technicians use the following steps to make impression castings:

1. The footwear or tire impression is thoroughly photographed using proper scale.
2. The impression is recorded with labels and a sketch.
3. Any foreign objects are removed and water is siphoned.
4. A wood or cardboard frame is used to build a retaining wall.
5. A cast is made of the total circumference of the tires or footwear as controls.
6. The casting is reinforced with wire or twigs.

Tool Marks

Tools are often used in the commission of crimes, such as for breaking into a residence or business. These tools leave imprints or impressions on surfaces, and these marks can be compared to the tool. Tool marks are commonly found in burglary and criminal mischief offenses. The tool or object may break during the commission of the crime so the surrounding area and debris are carefully checked for parts or fragments of tools.

Trace material can be transferred between the tool and tool mark surface. For example, paint from the surface of a window can be transferred to a pry bar. Paint from a pry bar can be transferred to the window. The tool mark is photographed and sketched prior to the collection process. In many cases, it is necessary for the crime scene technician to remove the tool mark and submit it to the laboratory. It is common for complete doors, windows, and other large items to be removed, protected, sealed, and sent in their entirety to the laboratory for analysis.

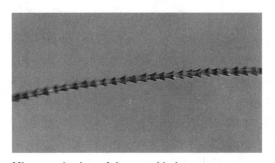

Microscopic view of damaged hair

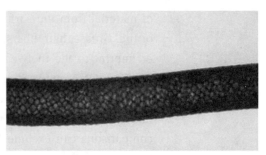

Microscopic view of raised cuticle hair

Hair

Human hair is found everywhere. The physical characteristics of hair can be described using color, width, morphology, length, curl, and a variety of other microscopic characteristics. These characteristics are compared microscopically between the known control (K) sample and the unknown hair (Q) collected at the scene. The process of comparing the questioned human hair (Q) to known human hairs (K) using comparison microscopes has been performed for years in the forensic community.

The collection of a representative control sample from a victim or suspect is a challenge in hair comparisons. At least 25 to 50 control hairs are needed to establish a baseline of physical characteristics in order to make the comparison to unknown hair samples. Attempts to compare hair samples with less than 25 to 50 control hairs will lessen the significance of the resulting expert opinion.

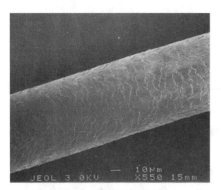

Microscopic view of healthy hair

The growth of DNA technology has impacted microscopic hair comparison. Nuclear DNA analysis of a hair root or mitochondrial DNA analysis of the hair shaft can result in a more definitive opinion than microscopic comparison. DNA analysis can categorically exclude the unknown hair as being the same as the known exemplar. As a result, some laboratories now only microscopically screen hair to determine its racial origin or whether it is suitable for nuclear DNA analysis or mitochondrial DNA shaft analysis. The replacement of more tedious microscopic hair comparisons

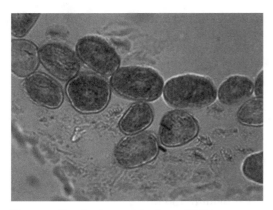

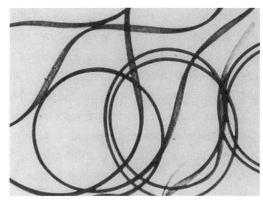

Cross-sectional microscopic view of hair   Showing a different texture of hair

with DNA analysis has resulted in the reassignment of forensic personnel from hair comparison units to other units in the laboratory.

Different types of human hair are collected and analyzed. Scalp, limb, body, and pubic hair are four common types of hair collected. Scalp hairs are collected to represent the total area of the scalp. Representative samples of scalp hair include 5 to 10 hairs from the top, left, right, front, and back of the scalp. The hair must be collected by combing and pulling the hairs, not by cutting. The hairs are then placed in paper envelopes, labeled, sealed, and sent to the laboratory for comparison.

Toxicology Specimens

Samples of the deceased victim's body are collected at the autopsy and submitted to the laboratory for analysis. In most cases, this is done when the cause of death is in question. In these cases, the medical examiner cannot determine the cause of death or needs more information to support her medical opinion. Urine, blood, and hair are also analyzed from living subjects to determine if they were driving while intoxicated from alcohol, or driving while impaired by drugs. Urine, blood, and hair may also be collected for drug abuse testing in the workplace.

Physiological fluids and tissue samples are routinely collected at the autopsy for toxicology analysis. These include blood, urine, stomach contents, bile, liver, kidney, brain, vitreous humor, and hair. These samples are analyzed for controlled substances, alcohol, prescription abuse, and poisons that may have caused death or impairment in the victim. The toxicology laboratory can detect very small amounts of compounds in the human body (in nanograms, or 1/1,000,000,000 gram). The medical examiner and toxicologist work together to determine if the controlled substances or other chemicals were sufficient to cause impairment or death. Crime scene technicians, detectives, and the medical examiner all work together as a team to determine cause of death.

Controlled substances are also a major cause of accidental deaths. Drug addicts use street drugs that contain contaminants. The drug addict may not be aware that the drugs contain a lethal dosage or mixture of controlled substances. Accidental deaths due to drug overdoses become criminal when the drug supplier is prosecuted for providing the drugs to the user. The following samples are collected at an autopsy for analysis of controlled substances: blood, urine, vitreous humor, brain, liver, stomach contents, and excised tissue at the injection site.

Poisons can cause both accidental and criminal homicides. Examples of the variety of common poisons and the tissue samples needed for analyses are listed here:

Common Poisons		**Tissue Sample Needed**
Inhaled gases or vapors	→	Lung tissue
Lead poisoning	→	Rib bone
Arsenic	→	Scalp hair and toe or fingernails
Cyanide	→	Blood

The crime scene team will collect all prescriptions, remedies, and controlled substances at the crime or accident scene. These samples will be delivered to the laboratory for comparison to any substances found in the toxicology analyses.

Frequently Asked Questions

Q: *Do all forensic laboratories have experts in toxicology?*

A: Most forensic laboratories do not have a toxicology laboratory. In large metropolitan areas, the toxicology laboratory is located within the medical examiner's office.

Q: *Are drugs difficult to find in toxicology analyses?*

A: Some drugs are difficult to detect because the metabolic half-life of the drug in the human body is very short. The only remaining trace of the substance may be a one- or two-generation metabolite that is not controlled or capable of causing impairment. The medical examiner must then extrapolate and estimate the level of the parent–controlled substance.

CHAPTER 9

Evidence from the Autopsy

D eath can be defined simply as the state in which the heart ceases to beat and respiration of the lungs no longer occurs. Recent advancements in medicine and the means to artificially support life have impacted the definition of death. Terms such as clinical death and brain death are used to more fully assess if a person is no longer alive. The physician determines death and the death certificate registers cause of death. In general,

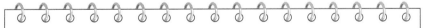

F. Lee Bailey's and H. Aronson's book, *The Defense Never Rests,* quotes the testimony of Dr. Milton Helpern, a celebrated forensic pathologist who was chief medical examiner of New York City from 1954 to 1973. Helpern testified at *State of New Jersey* v. *Carl Coppolino,* a trial in which Coppolino was accused of murdering the husband of his ex-mistress. "'In my opinion,' said Helpern, 'death resulted from the compression of the neck as indicated by this double fracture of the cricoid cartilage.'" (p. 260)

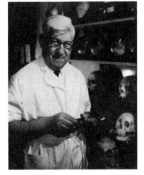

Milt Helpern, former chief medical examiner, New York City

if a person dies under a physician's care from a naturally occurring illness, the physician signs the death certificate. However, in cases of violent death, such as accidents, suicides or homicides, suspicious deaths, sudden and unexpected deaths, or deaths without a physician in attendance, the death becomes a medicolegal case. The term *medicolegal* implies the marriage between law and medicine. A forensic autopsy or postmortem examination is conducted in cases of medicolegal deaths.

Coroner's System versus Medical Examiner's System

Two medicolegal systems concern death investigation in the United States: the coroner's system and the medical examiner's system. The coroner's system has origins in Great Britain. The term *coroner* derives from *crowner,* and the original establishment of the coroner's office came from the King of England in the 10th century. The coroner is an elected official who makes rulings as to the cause and manner of death. In some jurisdictions in the United States, the coroner is not required to be a physician. For

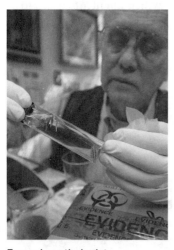

example, it is not uncommon for the coroner to be a local funeral home director or other nonmedical citizen of that county. In some locales, there are mandates that the coroner be a physician, but not necessarily a pathologist. There are consequences to this system. For example, deaths may be mishandled, evidence obliterated, and homicides mistakenly ruled as suicides, accidents, or even natural deaths.

The subspecialty of forensic pathology was established in 1959. Forensic pathologists complete advanced training including a bachelor's degree, medical school, a multi-

Forensic pathologist

year residency in pathology, and an additional fellowship in forensic pathology. The specialized training that a forensic pathologist receives is several orders of magnitude beyond the training that a family physician or a surgeon receives.

When an autopsy is requested in a hospital, it is done under the consent of the next of kin. A pathologist on staff at the hospital will perform the postmortem examination. It is not uncommon for the coroner to request that a hospital pathologist conduct a medicolegal autopsy. The pathologist must understand both the medical and legal skills needed, such as assessment of the trauma associated with unnatural death as well as the ability to clearly present findings to a jury in a court of law. These skills typically go beyond the scope of training that a hospital pathologist routinely receives.

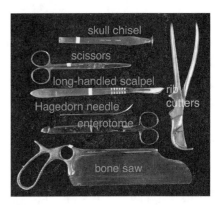

Autopsy tools

The concept of the medical examiner was first established in Massachusetts in 1877. By 1918, New York City had evolved to the point of the current structure of the medical examiner system in the United States. Dr. Milton Helpern (1902–1977) further developed the medical examiner system by establishing a modern facility for the scientific, educational, and investigative resources to conduct medicolegal autopsies and death investigations thoroughly. This included a forensic science laboratory to help determine cause and manner of death. Under the direction of the chief medical examiner, medicolegal deaths and investigations are managed and conducted by trained forensic pathologists. Both the coroner's system and the medical examiner's system currently exist in the United States. Some states have both medical examiner's and coroner's systems in place.

The Death Certificate: Cause and Manner of Death

Cause of death is the injury or disease that results in the person dying. Examples include a gunshot wound to the head or coronary atherosclerosis. It is not uncommon for a physician to mistakenly write cardiac arrest or cardiopulmonary arrest on a death certificate as the cause of death. Although these are simple definitions, they do not represent the *cause* of death, but are the *mechanisms* of death. Using the example of a gunshot wound, the mechanism of death might be hemorrhage resulting in exsanguination causing cardiac arrest. However, actual cause of death is still the gunshot wound.

The manner of death is how the cause of death came about. In the example of a gunshot wound, the manner of death could be ruled a homicide, indicating that someone other than the decedent fired the fatal shot. It could be ruled a suicide, indicating that the decedent shot himself. It could be ruled accidental, which could indicate that either the decedent or another individual was responsible for the weapon's discharge, but there was no intent to cause a fatality or harm. In cases involving accidental gunshot wounds, much care must be given to preserve the scene or to reconstruct the events surrounding the shooting to help ascertain the circumstances that differentiate an accident from a homicide or suicide.

There are five categories of manner of death. They are natural, accidental, suicide, homicide, and "could not be determined." The first four categories are relatively self-explanatory. "Could not be determined" is vague by comparison. A death is ruled undetermined when the circumstances surrounding the death are insufficient to make a determination. Often in these types of cases, the cause of death is listed as unknown with the manner ruled as undetermined. An undetermined ruling is not uncommon for deaths where all that is discovered of the body is advanced decomposition or skeletonized remains. If a decomposed body is discovered in a wooded area with a gunshot wound and there is no weapon in the vicinity, the likely manner of death would be homicide. However, if a gun was discovered near the body and the autopsy and scene investigation were not able to answer fundamental questions regarding the events that led up to how the death occurred, the coroner may choose to rule that the manner of death could not be determined. Was the decedent hunting and the weapon discharged accidentally? Could someone have shot the victim and left the gun behind to make it look like a suicide? Or was the individual suicidal without anyone having knowledge of this tendency? Perhaps the location of the gunshot wound may help eliminate these questions. For example, a self-inflicted gunshot wound to the back of the head is improbable.

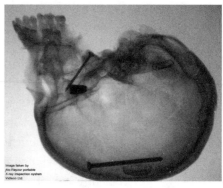

Human skull with foreign objects: How did those get there?

Information Assessed at the Autopsy

In addition to mechanism and manner of death, forensic autopsy attempts to answer the following:

- What is the time of death and the time interval between an injury(s) and death?
- What weapon (if any) was involved?
- What is the fatal wound?

- Was the body moved at the scene or to a secondary location?
- From what direction did the injury occur?
- Is there evidence of sexual assault?
- Were there any alcohol, drugs, or inhalants present in the body, and are they contributory to death?
- Are there any defense wounds present on the body to indicate a struggle with an assailant?

Various postmortem changes assist in predicting the approximate time of death or the postmortem interval. *Algor mortis* or postmortem cooling can be used to ascertain the time of death. The temperature of the body when it is discovered is recorded and compared to the ambient temperature of the environment the body is found in. Controlled studies have been conducted and are used as models for assessing temperature as a prediction for postmortem interval. On average, a body cools 1.5 to 2.5 degrees Farenheit per hour during the first hours up to 12 hours after death, with additional slowing to about one degree Farenheit for the next 12 to 18 hours. Multiple variables affect prediction of time of death using body temperature, such as certain drugs present in the body at the time of death, ambient temperatures warmer than body temperature, and the health of the individual at the time of death.

Livor mortis, or lividity, is the discoloration caused by the blood settling or pooling in the body after death. This occurs as a consequence of gravity—blood pools to the lower areas of the body. In the supine position, blood settles in the back, buttocks, and back of the legs, causing a purplish-blue color to develop. During early stages of *livor mortis,* if the pigmented areas are subject to compression with the thumb of the investigator, the skin will blanch or displace. After 8 to 12 hours the blood will coagulate in the vessels or diffuse into body tissues and this blanching will not occur. This is known as *fixed lividity.* Observation of fixed lividity patterns on the body may indicate that a body has been repositioned or that something has been removed from the scene that was pressing into the body. If lividity is not in the fixed state, the forensic pathologist can estimate that time of death occurred less than 12 hours previously. The forensic pathologist can also use the color of the lividity to aid in determining cause of death. In normal lividity, the color is bluish purple. In cases where carbon monoxide poisoning has occurred, lividity may be more cherry red in color.

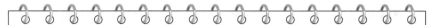

A recent child abuse homicide case demonstrates the importance of observing lividity. A young girl was admitted to the hospital dead on arrival (DOA). With no known existing medical conditions, her death became a coroner's case. At the morgue, there were no external findings. After 24 hours, the body revealed lividity patterns consistent with being in a prone position. Further observation revealed pressure points consistent with a handprint on the back of the neck. The case was ruled a homicide with cause of death as suffocation. Lividity findings were consistent with the girl being forcibly held down from the back of her neck and head as a consequence of child abuse.

Postmortem rigidity, or *rigor mortis,* is muscular stiffening that occurs in dead tissue as a result of the depletion of adensine triphosphate (ATP). Once death has occurred, metabolic activity does not stop completely in the muscle cells. There is a diminishing of activity that causes an increase in cellular acidity, resulting in a chemical fixation of cellular proteins. Initially after death, the body becomes very pliable. This flaccidness is soon followed by rigidity, fixing the joints in place. *Rigor mortis* develops in all of the muscles but first appears in the smaller muscles of the jaw. Temperature influences the rate at which *rigor mortis* begins and recedes. Increased temperatures may speed up the process. In ambient temperatures, *rigor mortis* typically begins to develop within the first hour of death; it is complete within 12 hours. This state remains about 12 hours, and then rigidity starts to recede, progressing in a reverse fashion over the course of an additional 12 hours. Age, muscle mass, and the presence of certain drugs in the body influence the rate and development of *rigor mortis.*

The contents of the stomach and the degree of digestion can also help determine the postmortem interval. If a missing person was last seen eating pepperoni pizza and three days later his body is discovered abandoned in a dumpster as a victim of homicide, the finding of particulate matter consistent with pepperoni pizza in the stomach may help place the time of death. Finding digested remains of the last meal consistent with activities that the victim was last observed engaged in, aids the investigation into events leading up to the death.

Degree of decomposition is also used as an indicator to estimate postmortem interval, but to a lesser degree than the above methods. While lividity and *rigor mortis* allow for time of death estimates in *hours,* degree of decomposition may involve estimates in *weeks* or *months,* depending on environmental conditions where the body was located.

Decomposition is the degradation or breakdown of the body. The process begins once death occurs and progresses until skeletonization is achieved, unless intervention slows the rate of decomposition. Intervention can be as simple as refrigeration or long term in the case of embalming. Whatever the means, intervention will not completely stop the decay process. Decomposition is achieved by both internal and external means. Internally, the body begins *autolysis,* where the cells of the body disintegrate, releasing enzymes that begin to break down organs and tissues. External forces begin the anaerobic process of putrefaction, where bacteria and other microorganisms release enzymes that decompose tissue. Some bacteria is found internally such as in the intestines. Putrefaction often produces methane gas as a by-product of the catabolism of body tissues. Certain variables can affect the rate of decomposition and accelerate or decelerate the process. Ambient temperature, access to insects, burial depth, rodent or other carnivore activity, trauma such as laceration or crushing, and humidity and aridity are variables that have a great effect on decomposition. Other variables have a lesser effect on the rate of decomposition. These include rainfall amount, body size and weight, degree of embalming, the type of clothing worn, and location and surface on which the body was placed.

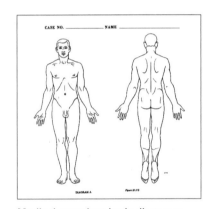

Medical examiner body diagrams

Dissection of the Forensic Autopsy

The forensic autopsy consists of the identification of the body, and includes tagging, measuring, weighing, and often x-raying the body, photographing the body, external examination of injuries, scars, and wounds, the dissection and internal examination of the body, toxicology studies of body fluids and tissues, and finally, the issuance of a death certificate complete with the cause and manner of death.

Identification of the body may be as simple as a visual identification in comparison with a driver's license or by a family member or friend.

Ohio Department of Health
VITAL STATISTICS
CERTIFICATE OF DEATH

Ohio death certificate

However, if the body cannot be identified by these means due to advanced decomposition or the nature of the injuries then additional avenues are pursued. Fingerprint comparisons, DNA testing, odontology comparisons between postmortem dental and antemortem dental X-rays, and radiographic comparisons of fractures with those observed healed on postmortem X-rays, can all be used to provide identification. Finding scars consistent with past surgical procedures or injuries and tattoos that the decedent was known to have also aid in identification.

Findings from external examination of the body are documented as the body is received into the morgue. All clothing, including the contents of pockets or accompanying bags, is recorded in the pathologist's notes. Photographs are taken depicting the body as received. Any scars, tattoos, or injuries are documented, as is height, weight, hair and eye color, and general condition of the body. X-rays may be done, especially in cases of gunshot wounds where it is necessary to determine the bullet tract and recover the projectile for evidentiary purposes. Any fractures are noted and diagrammed as part of the documentation process. For gunshot wounds, exit and entrance wounds are carefully examined and measured. Soot or abrasion near and around the entrance wound may indicate close contact with the barrel of the weapon at the time it was fired. Evidence of soot or gunpowder stippling near the entrance wound can indicate an intermediate range of the gun during firing. Gunshot entrance wounds are often irregular and can show varying characteristics dependent on the trajectory of the shot, body position, clothing or items worn on the body, and the type of ammunition used.

Body diagram with notes

In cases of violent death, the hands are typically bagged in paper sacks at the crime scene and remain encased until the pathologist begins the external examination of the hands in the morgue. The hands and fingernails are meticulously examined for wounds and breakage of the nails as this could indicate that the victim struggled with the attacker. Fingernails are often collected because the victim may have scratched the attacker, and the perpetrator's DNA might be under the victim's fingernails. Other evidence that can be recovered from the victim's hands include hair, fiber, and powder residue. The identification of gunpowder residue on the hands can help discern suicide from homicidal deaths in cases where manner of death is ambiguous. However, the absence of gunpowder residue on the hands does not eliminate suicide as the manner of death. Other implements such as toes or sticks can be used to pull the trigger on a weapon, especially rifles which are longer barreled, and when ergonomics prevents a finger from activating the trigger. Fingerprinting is done *after* the pathologist has completed the external examination and evidence is collected.

The external examination may involve swabbing body orifices such as oral, vaginal, and anal cavities. These may provide evidence, such as semen left behind by the perpetrator in cases of sexual assault. The eyes (especially inside the lower and upper eyelids) and the mouth mucosa should be examined for tiny pinpoint hemorrhages. These may indicate strangling, choking, or suffocation due to the increased blood pressure exerted on the head from asphyxia trauma.

Internal examination of the body involves the evisceration of body cavities. This procedure begins with a "Y" incision, so named because it runs from shoulder to shoulder, above the breasts, and down the sternum extending along the midline of the body and ending at the pubis, similar in shape to the letter Y. The skin is reflected back from the rib cage and the ribs are cut on either side, typically with a saw; the rib plate, including the sternum, is removed. This allows the neck area and chest cavity to be exposed.

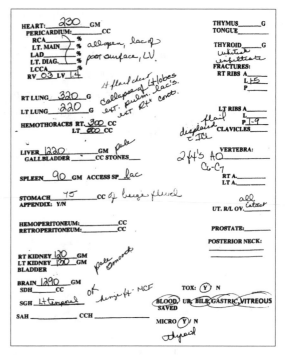

Autopsy notes

The neck organs, heart, and lungs will be visible. Any evidence of trauma is ascertained and noted prior to the removal of these organs. Careful examination of the neck may reveal evidence of manual strangulation (as mentioned earlier in Dr. Helpern's testimony), ligature impressions from hanging-type asphyxia deaths, and/or bruising consistent with trauma. Any blood or fluid found in the chest cavity is measured and a sample of blood is taken from the heart for toxicology. It is not unusual for the neck organs (trachea, esophagus, and thyroid gland), the heart, and the lungs to be removed together. This allows the pathologist to dissect these organs on a cutting surface, providing a closer examination. The nature of the case dictates the best type of removal procedure. Preservation of evidence and proper documentation of the trauma facilitates examination of wounds and tracing of wound tracts. The tongue may be removed along with the neck organs to allow examination of evidence of trauma.

Following the midline incision to the abdominal and pelvic cavities, this area is assessed. Any trauma or fluid observed is documented. Urine is collected from the bladder for toxicology studies. The abdominal organs are typically removed together; however, the spleen, liver, and kidneys (along with the adrenal glands) can be removed separately and the remaining digestive organs with the remaining genitourinary organs can be removed together. The testicles can be removed from the scrotum and examined either internally through the pelvic cavity or externally through an incision in the scrotum. Regardless of how they are removed, the organs are thoroughly examined and dissected. In addition, stomach contents are measured and examined. It is not uncommon for a portion of the stomach contents to be submitted for toxicology studies.

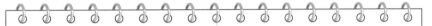

In the following case, the use of luminol to detect blood, coupled with the medicolegal exam of the victim, disproved the suspect's alibi. A woman was found dead in a field miles from her home. She had been reported missing by her husband days earlier. At autopsy, multiple blunt force trauma wounds with lacerations were observed on her head and torso. The cause of death was blunt force trauma to the head and the manner was determined to be homicide. At the home the couple shared, multiple latent bloodstains were observed when luminol was used in the bathroom. The husband stated that he had cleaned up blood from his wife's menstrual period. At autopsy, a corpus luteum was observed in the ovary. This finding placed the woman at the midpoint or ovulation of her menstrual cycle, thus negating the husband's story that the blood was a consequence of menstruation. The husband then confessed to beating his wife in the head and body until she died and then dumping her body in the field.

The final area typically examined during the internal examination is the head and brain. An incision is made behind the ear, from ear to ear, and the scalp is carefully reflected back, peeling it forward and away from the skull. A saw is used to cut the skull. This instrument is similar to the saw used to remove casts from arms and legs. Once an opening is created in the skull, the brain is examined and any blood or hemorrhage is noted before the organ is removed. The brain is carefully examined. Depending on the nature of death, a neuropathologist specializing in the injury and disease states of the brain, may be employed for both the gross and the microscopic examination of the brain.

The final report summarizes all of the findings noted during the course of the autopsy. It includes internal, external, and microscopic examinations performed on the body. During the course of the autopsy, each organ that is removed is weighed and that weight is recorded as part of the autopsy report. Sections or cuttings from organs or tissues may be taken at the discretion of the pathologist. These can be used in microscopic studies that allow evaluation of cellular changes that assist in the diagnosis of disease states. All fluid volumes are noted in the autopsy report as is any trauma observed. Any irregularities are mentioned. Alternatively, the organ is deemed unremarkable, indicating that it is normal in size, shape, and function without evidence of trauma or malady. Autopsy reports, photographs, microscopic slides, and any notes recorded by the forensic pathologist are maintained as part of the case file.

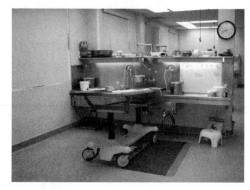

Autopsy suite

At the conclusion of the autopsy, all organs are returned to the body and the body is sutured. In cases where the body will be embalmed, preservative agents will be admixed with the organs. By returning the organs to the body cavity, they are available for reexamination or a subsequent autopsy. Should the need arise, the body is exhumed from its grave.

Toxicology

Toxicology studies are often the determining factor for both the cause and manner of death. Drug screens identify the type of substance as well as postmortem concentration in the fluids tested. In addition to blood, urine,

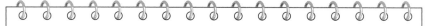

The body of an elderly man was exhumed after his death, which was believed to be of natural causes. His wife had received a notice that his artificial heart valve had been demonstrated to be defective in other recipients. The wife questioned the reliability of the heart valve product and she coordinated the exhumation of her husband's body. At autopsy, the heart valve was intact and appeared to have been functioning properly. No additional gross evidence was found to explain his death. The nasal cavities were swabbed for toxicology and a high level of cocaine and its metabolites were detected. The wife corroborated that the husband had used cocaine recreationally. The cause of death was determined to be acute cocaine intoxication and the death was ruled accidental.

and the stomach contents, bile and vitreous fluid are often collected at autopsy and submitted for toxicology. In cases where the body is decomposed, muscle tissue can be used. Any tissue in the body can be sent for toxicology, but typically the blood, urine, and vitreous fluid offer the most value. Studies include routine screening for alcohol concentration and drugs of abuse, such as cocaine, heroin, methamphetamine, and marijuana. Scientists also perform an analysis for carbon monoxide concentration and heavy metals and poisons, such as lead, arsenic, and cyanide.

Public Safety

A medicolegal autopsy is needed in cases of homicide and suicide. The autopsy plays a role in public safety when it reveals contrary findings in deaths believed to be natural or accidental. Autopsy also helps detect environmental and mechanical hazards in deaths due to occupational risks, such as asbestos, pesticide poisoning, or ineffective safety procedures. In automobile accidents, the autopsy can evaluate the effectiveness of seat belts and air bags, providing information that assists manufacturers in the design of safer restraints.

Frequently Asked Questions

Q: *What types of court cases are forensic pathologists involved in?*

A: In addition to testifying in criminal court, the forensic pathologist may be called upon to testify in civil litigations due to cases involving safety negligence.

Q: *What is the length of time that autopsy documentation is maintained?*

A: Typically, autopsy files are retained indefinitely.

Q: *Do the crime scene team members assist at autopsies?*

A: Yes, detectives and crime scene technicians routinely go to autopsies to assist in sample collection.

Laura Lake Residence, 159 Walnut Street, Metroland, New York

Dr. Ali Kumar was appointed by the mayor five years ago to be Metro County's first full-time medical examiner. As Metroland's population approached 2 million, the annual number of homicides warranted a full-time medical examiner to replace part-time consultants. Dr. Kumar and a laboratory technician perform a full autopsy on the victim, Laura Lake. The cause of death is loss of blood due to trauma on the head from a blunt instrument. There is no evidence of sexual assault. Wounds on both hands are consistent with defensive behavior during the assault. There are no fibers, fingerprints, or other trace evidence found amongst the clothing of the victim or upon the body. Unfortunately, Dr. Kumar can find no corroborative evidence to assist the detectives handling the homicide investigation.

CHAPTER 10

Processing a Vehicle

M otor vehicles are a significant source of evidence for a variety of cases.

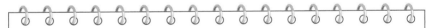

MARK'S STORY

One day before going on patrol, I mentioned to my sergeant and mentor that I wished we had a better strategy to find a particular burglar who was breaking into homes almost every night in an upscale neighborhood. He said, "Hey kid, go to that neighborhood and stop some cars. A burglar needs a car to get around." We caught a burglar in possession of stolen property in his car that night by setting up checkpoints in the neighborhood.

Common sense can be directly applied to all crimes. All criminals need vehicles to get around. The next step is to apply Locard's principle to the motor vehicle. How can we find and compare the known Ks and questioned Qs when an automobile is used in the commission of a crime?

Minor vehicular accidents and other crimes in which vehicles are used are some of the best sources of evidence training for new crime scene personnel, because these types of investigations are more frequent and just as complex as burglary, assault, and homicide. The techniques of evidence collection and laboratory analysis are all the same, and these complex investigations provide a treasure trove of physical evidence. Just as important, the crime scene team and laboratory may be able to exclude how the accident happened. The evidence analysis may not support the statements provided by the driver(s) of the vehicles.

Several scenarios require that a vehicle be processed by crime scene personnel.

A One-Car Property Damage Accident

This type of incident provides an opportunity for a new crime scene technician to learn the basics of recognition, collection, and protection of evidence with proper packaging, seals, and chain of custody. These lesser offenses have no injuries or serious consequences; however, technicians apply all the steps for proper search, recognition, and collection of evidence. A minor property damage accident investigation determines what property the vehicle contacted to confirm the source of the property damage. For example, a vehicle may strike public or personal property and the case may proceed to the small claims court for damage payment. Evidentiary analyses may be necessary to confirm that the vehicle caused the property damage.

The known items of evidence or controls will be paint and the remaining broken pieces still attached to the automobile, such as parts of the grill or headlight lens. Physically matching these items to items left at the scene is very significant. The debris from the scene will contain the Qs and the vehicle will provide the Ks for comparison.

Personal Injury: Single or Multivehicle Accidents

The consequences of these types of accidents can be significant if there are multiple and serious injuries to the occupants of the vehicles. Criminal and civil litigation may often develop as claims with insurance agencies and against all parties in the appropriate court system. There may be a felony charge of vehicular assault against the driver of one of the vehicles. The occupants of the vehicles are often unable to recollect the sequence of events that led to the accident. Attorneys representing plaintiffs may not allow detailed statements from victims or suspects. Only the evidence can prove or disprove how the vehicles came into contact and potentially confirm the placement of the driver and passengers in the vehicles. The crime scene technician will most probably testify in criminal and civil court for these types of cases. In addition to the collection of evidence to verify the contact of vehicles, trace evidence will be collected from the interior of the vehicle to show occupant placement. Driver injuries usually leave trace amounts of biological material on the inside surfaces of the vehicle, and verify the location of the individual at the time of the collision.

The Ks and Qs to confirm the collision are collected the same way as the property damage accident. The Ks for the occupant placement are blood and hair samples from the occupants. The Qs are the blood and hair trace evidence collected from the interior surfaces of the vehicle.

Vehicular Homicide: Multivehicle or Pedestrian Accident

This is the most serious type of vehicular accident. It will require the skills of an experienced crime scene and accident reconstruction team. Criminal charges for these types of cases typically result in convictions and multiple-year sentences in state prison. The process of evidence collection in these serious cases—to verify the contact of vehicles and placement of individuals—is identical to the personal injury and property damage accidents.

Vehicle Used in the Commission of a Crime

A vehicle could be used to transport suspects to and from the crime scene. The vehicle may have been used to transport stolen property or narcotics. The vehicle itself may be the stolen property: There are often tool marks, fingerprints, and trace DNA found on specific places within the interior of a vehicle that were compromised to start the engine and steal the vehicle. A vehicle is also commonly used to transport the victim of a homicide from the crime scene to a burial or disposal site.

The Ks are the known items of clothing, hair, and blood from the victim or suspect. The Qs are the trace amounts of fiber, hair, and blood found in the vehicle.

Driver or Passenger Impaired with Alcohol, Prescribed Drugs, or Illegally Possessed Controlled Substances

All police agencies train officers in methods to determine if a driver of a vehicle is impaired by alcohol or drugs. There also may be drugs or prescriptions found in the possession of the driver or in the vehicle. If observations and evidence substantiate the impairment of a driver, the detective or patrol officer will follow procedure and obtain a court order to obtain a blood and urine sample from the driver of the vehicle in the accident. The blood or urine is then submitted to the laboratory for analyses.

The Ks in this type of investigation are known controlled substances and prescriptions that are part of the controlled substance inventory in the toxicology section of the laboratory. The Qs are the trace amounts of these substances that may be found in the blood, tissues, or urine through instrumental analyses. The toxicology and controlled substance section of the laboratory can detect very small amounts of any compound (e.g., nanograms, or 1/1,000,000,000 gram).

Vehicular System Failure Analysis and Specialized Search

There also may be an engineering analysis to include or exclude vehicular mechanical failures. For example, there may have been a brake, steering, or tire failure. The driver may have been impaired from an exhaust system leak that permeated the interior with carbon dioxide. The carbon dioxide can cause drowsiness of the driver and lead to an accident. Some forensic laboratories have dedicated space for a forensic garage. The garage provides all the space and tools needed to properly process a vehicle for trace evidence. A vehicle lift is often used to raise the vehicle in a safe manner to allow forensic scientists to process the undercarriage for trace evidence. Blood, hair, other trace evidence, and drugs are often found behind panels and in hidden compartments. The crime scene team and professional automobile mechanic may be required to partially dismantle the vehicle to thoroughly examine it for all types of evidence.

Vehicular assault and homicide cases can lead to felony convictions and a sentence of confinement in prison for the driver. These types of cases result in more litigation and criminal prosecutions as the community becomes less tolerant of impaired driving. Crime scene personnel often work closely as a team with accident reconstruction personnel and they process the accident scene together. Evidence at the scene will help investigators determine how the accident happened and who was driving. Vehicular hit-and-run cases are classic examples of the Locard principle. How can we find trace evidence from the vehicle on the victim and trace evidence from the victim on the vehicle?

Searching a Vehicle

The two major approaches to processing a vehicle are the interior and exterior search. The crime scene team must consult with the district attorney to determine if a search warrant is needed.

Vehicle Interior

Team members use labels to divide the interior of the vehicle into distinct areas. For example, the back of the driver's seat is A, the bench seat for the driver is B, the floor driver side is C, etc. Sketches and photographs are just as important in processing a vehicle as in any other type of crime scene. The crime scene team will need to confirm the placement of individuals in the vehicle. For example, who was the driver of the vehicle at the time of the accident? Who was in the backseat or passenger's seat? Also, the team must be alert for any medications or controlled substances that may have caused impairment of the driver. It is common for victims and suspects to be represented by attorneys and to refuse all statements. An investigator may proceed as there are no statements at this stage of the investigation. The location and collection of evidence may end up being the only factor that can solve the case.

Vehicle Exterior

Crime scene personnel label areas on the outside of the vehicle in a similar way as the interior. The left fender is area H, the grill is area I, the right fender is area J, etc. A hit-and-run accident will require the crime scene team to collect known paint samples from the vehicle. These will be used to compare to questioned traces of paint found on the hit-and-run victim's clothing or second vehicle in a two-car accident. The team should consider collecting known samples from the damaged grill and headlight areas. Personnel must collect everything that may connect the vehicle to the incident.

Vehicular accidents also create a zone of debris on the roadway. This debris should be collected for analysis at the laboratory. The debris may support the fact that two vehicles actually did crash. Multiple vehicular accidents may be very complex to reconstruct. The debris on the roadway will enable the investigator to sort out the vehicle(s) involved in the accident(s) at the time of the collision. Clothes from a hit-and-run accident victim are potentially the most probative items of evidence. The crime scene team will go to the hospital or morgue and retrieve the clothing for examination at the laboratory. A close working relationship with emergency room and autopsy personnel is critical to the successful collection of this type of trace evidence. Technicians may also need to collect victim control samples of blood and hair at the hospital or morgue for comparison to trace evidence found at the vehicle involved in the incident.

Property damage, vehicular assault, and homicide accidents are investigated alone by a uniformed patrol officer of a police department. The police agency may even have an accident reconstruction team that will help the patrol officer investigate the accident with the use of surveying computer equipment. The multiple vehicle vehicular assault or homicide accident investigations are very intense and complex. The police, fire, and emergency personnel usually arrive within minutes of one another and must work as a team. Victims may need immediate medical attention. The patrol officer must remain calm and always remember safety, medical attention to the victims, and the Locard principle—"Recognize, collect, and protect the Ks and Qs."

Frequently Asked Questions

Q: *Does the crime scene team respond to most vehicular accidents?*

A: No. In most agencies the crime scene team is dedicated to criminal cases such as assaults and homicides. The patrol officer may single-handedly process a vehicular accident.

Q: *What is the most challenging part of the accident investigation?*

A: Time is of the essence. Victims may require medical attention. Vehicles may be on fire. The roadway may be closed and hundreds of vehicles may be stopped in traffic. The accident investigation may need to be completed within hours.

Q: *What is the relationship between patrol officer and crime scene personnel?*

A: The patrol officer has a close relationship with crime scene personnel and the laboratory. Knowledge of the techniques used by the crime scene team and laboratory will provide the patrol officer with tools that will allow him to solve the most complex cases with physical evidence.

Laura Lake Residence
Metroland, New York

Sam Livingston's vehicle is taken to the garage at the forensic laboratory and dismantled. The seats, interior molding, and carpeting are all removed and processed for trace evidence, such as blood and fibers, from the victim, Laura Lake. Forensic scientists work side by side with auto mechanics and collect hundreds of samples for analysis in the lab. The hairs and fibers found in the vehicle are compared to known samples from the victim with negative results.

CRIME SCENE

CHAPTER 11

Introduction to Evidence Receiving: Drug Chemistry

The Laboratory Evidence Receiving Unit

Evidence receiving is indisputably one of the most important sections of the forensic science laboratory. Here, all evidence enters and leaves the lab. "Customers" include patrol officers, detectives, prosecutors, and medical examiners. These customers interact with evidence receiving to submit, retrieve, and determine the status of evidence. Evidence receiving is one of the major gateways to the scientific expertise and technology that can make or break a case in the criminal justice community.

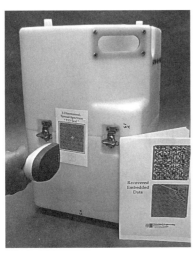

Bar codes are used for inventory and chain of custody

Evidence receiving is the first human contact that a police officer or member of the crime scene team has with the lab. At this entry point, the main concern is to ensure that evidence is properly packaged, labeled, and sealed, and that accurate submission forms accompany the evidence. Evidence receiving is where chain of custody starts for the laboratory and improperly packaged evidence may be rejected.

Routine evidence is usually packaged in boxes or plastic containers. These containers must be sealed and labeled properly. A proper seal prevents evidence loss and contamination. The seal must also be compromised when opening the evidence container. Most agencies use two-inch packing tape with unique logos for their

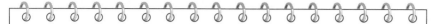

MARK'S STORY

Troopers are trained on proper methods to collect and handle evidence, with many lecture hours devoted to the services available at the lab. But the reality is that patrol officers are apprehensive about collecting and submitting evidence. They do not want to make a mistake and compromise the case in any way.

Very early in my career, I worked as a trooper in a small barracks in downstate New York. The barracks were literally across the parking lot from a regional forensic laboratory operated by the New York State Police. One day I sat down for a cup of coffee with the laboratory director and assistant director, a retired forensic scientist from the New York City Crime Lab. I received a realistic job preview of the forensic disciplines, including how evidence is collected, preserved, protected, and submitted for processing. I learned how the lab operates to serve the criminal justice community. These experts were the first of many professional mentors throughout my career. Professional networks between the lab, law enforcement, and the courts are critical to provide the highest quality forensic services.

agency and a color scheme for different types of evidence. Specialized evidence tampering tape is also available. This tape is very fragile and serrated for use with unique items packaged in small containers or envelopes. All seals are initialed and dated to show when and who made the seal. A submission form is completed by the person submitting the evidence; the form contains specific information needed for the laboratory to begin analysis. The submission form contains unique case numbers, the agency name, a description of the crime, inventory of evidence, and victim and suspect names. Most important in this process is to ensure an accurate inventory. Evidence receiving personnel check the inventory to make sure it corresponds exactly with the submission form. Any discrepancies in inventory, packaging, labeling, and sealing must be resolved and corrected before the evidence is accepted in the laboratory.

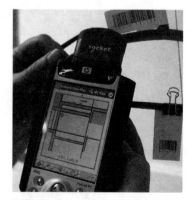

Bar code provides unique case identifier

Chain of custody for the laboratory begins when evidence receiving personnel accept the evidence as properly packaged, sealed, and labeled with an accurate and complete inventory. Traditionally, this was done with bound logbooks in which the submitter signs in to the laboratory and is given the next sequential laboratory case number. The unique laboratory case number is then written on all of the evidence containers. The evidence is then stored in designated storage rooms that have limited access and enhanced security. Designated storage rooms and authorized personnel are components of the chain of custody. Receipt or transfer logbooks are used to track evidence flow within the laboratory. Chain of custody evidence transactions must be documented at the time of transfer.

The traditional logbooks and receipts for the chain of custody process have been replaced in most laboratories by a laboratory information management system (LIMS). LIMS uses computer bar code tracking systems and document management systems in the laboratory. Some laboratories have expanded LIMS and initiate the bar code system at the crime scene. Evidence receiving personnel enter unique case information to generate bar codes and affix them to all items within the case. The bar codes are then scanned at all chain of custody transaction points within the laboratory. LIMS provides an accurate inventory for all evidence storage locations and evidence undergoing analyses.

Some types of evidence require special handling and storage. Biological (such as blood and sexual assault kits) and toxicology evidence must be refrigerated to prevent biodegradation. Firearms must be examined and confirmed to be in the "safe and unloaded" condition. Controlled substances require an accurate count of all pills, capsules, and paraphernalia.

Many laboratories assign new scientists to evidence receiving as a critical component of training. The lessons learned in chain of custody, evidence handling, security, and storage provide a fundamental understanding of the entire process. Firsthand knowledge of the evidence handling process enables forensic scientists to testify with authority and confidence.

Drug Section

The drug section in the forensic laboratory is often called "controlled substances" or "chemistry." This section handles, by far, the largest number of cases and items submitted to the laboratory. There are limitless numbers and types of powders, capsules, liquids, solids, paraphernalia, and plant material that contain controlled substances.

The definitions of controlled substances are found in state and federal penal laws. These drugs have been found to be addictive and cause physical and mental impairment. Many of these compounds can be legally obtained through a medical prescription. Federal and state laws define the provisions of the controlled substance violations. For example, the penal law of New York State clearly defines all the terms in which controlled substances are illegal in the state. These compounds are divided into two major sections of law:

1. The possession of controlled substances, and
2. The sale of controlled substances

The main web portal for the laws of New York provides access to more detail: *http://public.leginfo.state.ny.us/menugetf.cgi.*

Penal law offenses are generally more severe for the sale of controlled substances, as compared to the possession of controlled substances. The possession and sale offenses are further defined by amounts (quantity) and purity (quality) of the controlled substance. The terms "aggregate weight" and "pure weight" are also used to define the penal law charges in many jurisdictions. The quantity and quality of the drugs determine the "cutoffs" or threshold amount of drugs needed to sustain a charge.

The forensic scientist must perform two main tasks:

1. Analyze an unknown substance and confirm the presence of a controlled substance through a multitechnique molecular confirmation (qualitative procedure), and
2. Determine the pure weight of the substance (quantitative procedure) relative to what the penal law charge requires

For example, a kilogram of cocaine may be submitted as a "possession" case. The penal law may only require the confirmation of cocaine being present (qualitative procedure to determine the presence of a compound through multitechnique molecular confirmation) and the aggregate weight. An analytical balance would be used to weigh the kilogram of cocaine without any packaging to determine the exact weight. A more serious penal law section may require a pure weight. Quantitative analysis would be performed to determine the purity of the cocaine. If the purity was 80 percent, then the reported pure weight would be accurately defined, limited by the sensitivities and confidence or uncertainty levels of the method, as approximately 800 grams. These measurements are critical for the prosecutor to charge the defendant with the highest charge defined in penal law. Instrument sensitivities, detection limits, and uncertainty of measurements are critical knowledge for the forensic scientist.

The submitting police officer will classify the case as a "sale" or "possession" criminal investigation to assist the laboratory in selecting appropriate analyses to support the prosecution of the offense. Many "sale" criminal cases are sequential "buys" from the same suspect. LIMS is used to link these cases. Laboratory supervisors may assign one chemist to a string of buys to limit the number of staff testifying in the case.

The packaging of drug cases may also require processing for latent fingerprints. In these cases, LIMS makes a case assignment for the latent fingerprint unit. Some laboratories, such as the Drug Enforcement Administration (DEA), have latent fingerprint examiners within the drug lab in order to expedite the processing of drug packaging for latent fin-

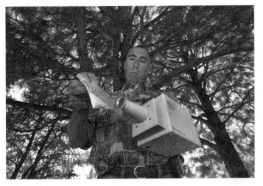

Drug detection electron microscope

gerprints. Forensic scientists and latent print examiners work as a team to open the evidence and separate the packaging from the drug contents.

Street drugs are contaminated mixtures. It can be difficult to separate and confirm the presence and quantity of controlled substances. Research and academic laboratories are accustomed to using pure compounds purchased from major pharmaceutical laboratories. Forensic scientists purchase these pure compounds as known controls (K). However, unknown (Q) street samples contain all types of degraded by-products that result from clandestine laboratory methods and impurities. Forensic scientists use separation and presumptive testing techniques to eliminate noncontrolled substances, to ultimately isolate and confirm the presence of a controlled substance.

The Scientific Working Group for the Analysis of Siezed Drugs (SWGDRUG) recommends an analytical scheme, sampling plan (figure 11.1), and general process for forensic drug analyses. Laboratories follow these professional recommendations to apply the best combination of science and technology to the evidence.

Street drugs submitted to the laboratory are often in large bulk amounts, such as thousands of items of pills or tablets. It would take months for a forensic scientist to perform the qualitative and quantitative analyses

FIGURE 11.1 *Sampling Scheme—A Decision Flowchart*

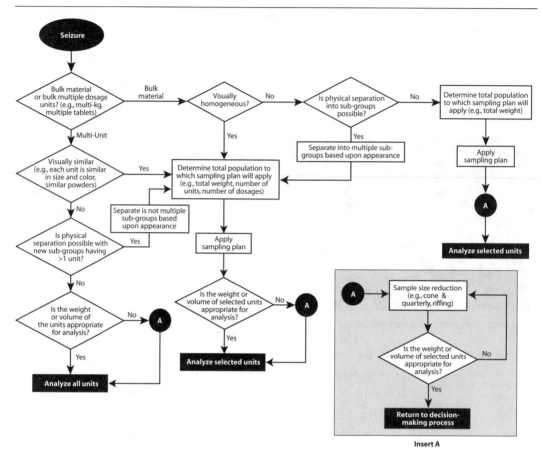

needed for each item. Laboratories work with the prosecutor to design a statistical sampling plan that projects the amount of analysis needed to support the highest charge in the penal law. The forensic scientist needs a strong background is statistics to testify in these types of cases.

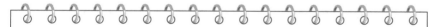

Techniques for the analysis of drug samples are classified into three categories based on their discriminating power. Table 11.1 provides examples of these techniques listed in order of decreasing discriminatory power, from A to C.

TABLE 11.1 *Categories of Analytical Techniques*

Category A	Category B	Category C
Infrared Spectroscopy	Capillary Electrophoresis	Color Tests
Mass Spectrometry	Gas Chromatography	Fluorescence Spectroscopy
Nuclear Magnetic Resonance Spectroscopy	Ion Mobility Spectrometry	Immunoassay
Raman Spectroscopy	Liquid Chromatography	Melting Point
	Microcrystalline Tests	Ultraviolet Spectroscopy
	Pharmaceutical Identifiers	
	Thin Layer Chromatography	

	Cannabis only:
	  Macroscopic Examination
	  Microscopic Examination	

3 Identification criteria

SWGDRUG recommends that laboratories adhere to the following minimum standards:

3.1 When a validated Category A technique is incorporated into an analytical scheme, then at least one other technique (from either Category A, B or C) shall be used.

3.1.1 This combination shall identify the specific drug present and shall preclude a false positive identification.

3.1.2 When sample size allows, the second technique should be applied on a separate sampling for quality assurance reasons. When sample size is limited, additional measures should be taken to assure that the results correspond to the correct sample.

3.1.3 All Category A techniques shall have data that are reviewable.

3.2 When a Category A technique is not used, then at least three different validated methods shall be employed.

3.2.1 These in combination shall demonstrate the identity of the specific drug present and shall preclude a false positive identification.

3.2.2 Two of the three methods shall be based on uncorrelated techniques from Category B.

3.2.3 A minimum of two separate samplings should be used in these three tests. When sample size is limited, additional measures should be taken to assure that the results correspond to the correct sample.

3.2.4 All Category B techniques shall have reviewable data.

3.3 For the use of any method to be considered of value, test results shall be considered "positive." While "negative" test results provide useful information for ruling out the presence of a particular drug or drug class, these results have no value toward establishing the forensic identification of a drug.

3.4 In cases where hyphenated techniques are used (e.g. gas chromatography-mass spectrometry, liquid chromatography-diode array ultraviolet spectroscopy), they will be considered as separate techniques provided that the results from each are used.

TABLE 11.1 *Categories of Analytical Techniques (continued)*

3.5	Cannabis exhibits tend to have characteristics that are visually recognizable. Macroscopic and microscopic examinations of cannabis will be considered, exceptionally, as uncorrelated techniques from Category B when observations include documented details of botanical features. Additional testing shall follow the scheme outlined in sections 3.1 or 3.2.
3.5.1	For exhibits of cannabis that lack sufficient observable macroscopic and microscopic botanical detail (e.g. extracts or residues), (delta-9-tetrahydrocannabinol (THC) or other cannabinoids shall be identified utilizing the principles set forth in sections 3.1 and 3.2.
3.6	An identification of botanical material may be made utilizing morphological characteristics alone, provided sufficient botanical features appropriate for identification are observed. Such examinations shall be made by analysts competent in botanical identifications. In this context botanical competence applies to those examiners recognized as professional botanists or those assessed to be competent by such. Identifications of chemical components contained in botanicals (mescaline, opiates, psilocin, etc.) should rely on principles of chemical identification.
3.7	Examples of reviewable data are: • printed spectra, chromatograms and photographs or photocopies of TLC plates • contemporaneous documented peer review for microcrystalline tests • reference to published data for pharmaceutical identifiers • recording of detailed descriptions of morphological characteristics for cannabis (only)

Source: Scientific Working Group for the Analysis of Seized Drugs (SWGDRUG) at *www.swgdrug.org/ Documents/SWGDRUG%20Recommendations.htm*

Frequently Asked Questions

Q: *What are the challenging aspects of being a forensic drug chemist?*

A: Forensic drug chemists face the daunting challenge of identifying trace amounts of controlled substances in a contaminated mixture of street drugs. This involves hypothesis testing with scientific data to confirm or exclude the presence of a controlled substance. This formidable challenge will test the education, analytical abilities, and analytical instruments used by the scientist.

Q: *What are the negative aspects of being a forensic drug chemist?*

A: Forensic drug chemists perform the same type of analyses every day. For example, most cases may involve cocaine, heroin, and marijuana. After several years, the forensic scientist will have seen most types of drugs and will need new challenges in learning instrumentation and techniques. Laboratories provide career enrichment and professional development activities to address issues that occur with routine work.

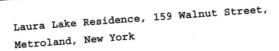

Laura Lake Residence, 159 Walnut Street,
Metroland, New York

Sam Livingston is now a suspect in the case. He has retained Howard Chapin, defense attorney, who has requested that the laboratory produce all documents related to the crime scene, evidence receiving section, and all laboratory analyses. He will assign staffers in his office to review all documentation to uncover any type of transactional errors or human errors in the chain of custody, sealing of evidence, inventory of all items of evidence, and laboratory analyses. A forensic expert in DNA and crime scene processing will be under contract to provide a technical review of all laboratory work performed for the Laura Lake homicide. Quality assurance manager Carol Lent will work closely with the police department's legal counsel and the district attorney to ensure all pertinent documents are properly disclosed in a timely manner to the defense. They do not want a mistrial due to lack of disclosure of probative documents.

CRIME SCENE

CHAPTER 12

Biology

Overview

Developments in forensic molecular biology have revolutionized forensic science. Forensic labs are inundated with requests for forensic biology cases due to the discriminating power of DNA technology. In a relatively short 20 years, traditional ABO blood typing methods have evolved to DNA analysis, with high certainties of identity. Early methods of ABO and electrophoresis could categorically exclude a suspect but had little value for determining positive identification. The newest DNA analysis method—multiplex polymerase chain reaction short tandem repeat (PCR-STR)—is capable of producing sole source attribution probabilities of one in a trillion or more.

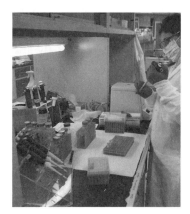

DNA scientist

The structure for the double-stranded DNA molecule was first described by Watson and Crick in the 1950s. Since then, basic research on DNA has led to the development and application of numerous state-of-the-art molecular identification technologies for the forensic community. DNA typing technology was first used successfully in a forensic laboratory in 1985 by Dr. Alec Jeffreys. Describing what he called "DNA fingerprinting,"

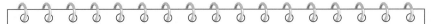

There are no limits to the possibilities for gathering DNA evidence. *Any* source of human physiological material provides potential evidence for a DNA profile. Detectives obtain DNA evidence in four ways: through data-banks, court orders, voluntary samples, or through abandonment. The Combined DNA Index System (CODIS) is a data bank legislated through state and federal law. Court orders are used to obtain samples from crime suspects. Voluntary samples are obtained from suspects and victims.

The most innovative samples are collected through abandonment. If a suspect leaves a coffee cup, cigarette butt, or other material in a public place, detectives can collect the item for DNA analysis. The widely successful Biotracks program in New York City targeted abandonment samples and the biological evidence collected at lesser criminal offenses, such as burglaries. Many burglaries and larcenies were solved, linking them to other similar crimes and even violent offenses.

Jeffreys recognized that certain regions of DNA contain repeats of the same sequences; these repeat regions vary in length in different individuals. Dr. Jeffreys used a molecular biology technique known as restriction fragment length polymorphism (RFLP) to compare molecules. In conjunction with the repeated sequences, or variable number of tandem repeats (VNTR), RFLP provided a very powerful tool for forensic DNA typing. However, the process was costly and time consuming, taking six to eight weeks to develop. In addition, the use of radioactive probes presented a safety hazard. There were other limitations, in that at least .05 micrograms of intact DNA was required to successfully analyze an RFLP-generated DNA profile.

In 1986, Kari Mullis developed a molecular DNA technique known as polymerase chain reaction (PCR). PCR revolutionized forensic DNA typing, because it allowed very small

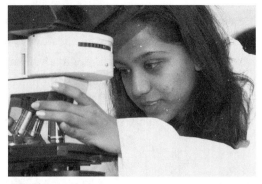

Microscopic visualization of evidence

amounts of DNA recovered from the crime scene to be amplified. Using this highly sensitive amplification technique, a DNA molecule is replicated many times. Each newly copied DNA molecule can serve as template

DNA in future cycles. In a three-hour run (28 cycles), millions of copies of specific target DNA can be produced. PCR technology meets the needs of the forensic crime lab, in that it is sensitive, safe, fast, robust, and economical.

Forensic labs continue to push the sensitivity threshold even lower by performing PCR amplification on select regions of the DNA molecule. A number of benefits arise as analytic techniques improve. These include high through-put potential and an overall decrease in turnaround time for DNA typing casework. Prior to improvements in STR-PCR technology, attempts to profile degraded DNA samples often produced inconclusive results. Forensic labs have had recent success obtaining profiles from fragmented and degraded DNA samples. Examples include disaster sites, such as those from TWA Flight 800, Swissair Flight 111, and the World Trade Center.

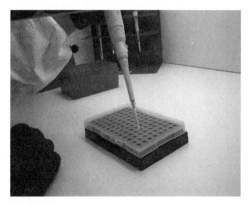

Pipetting DNA extractions

The forensic biology laboratory is divided into two sections, serology and DNA. The serology laboratory is the first section to open a biology case and begin analysis. The forensic scientist opens the seals of the case and checks the inventory of the evidence against the evidence submission form. Any discrepancies in the seals, packaging, or in additional or missing items will be resolved before beginning the analysis. Analyses of samples from victims and suspects must be separated by *time and space.* Contamination between the suspect's and victim's evidence negates future DNA comparison. The appropriate DNA standards and blank controls are also run concurrent with the items of evidence.

The serology laboratory screens all incoming evidence for human semen, blood, and saliva stains. Screening tests are designed to eliminate negative material from subsequent costly and time-consuming DNA analysis. A variety of presumptive screening chemical tests indicate the presence of human biological materials. Stains and liquids identified by these screening techniques are forwarded to the DNA unit for analysis.

TABLE 12.1 *Presumptive Test with Samples That Contain Blood and Ascorbic Acid*

Reagent	Blood Concentration in Samples (mL Blood/mL Solution)				
	A	B	C	D	E
0-Tolidine	+	+	+	−	−
Tetramethylbenzidine	+	+	+	+	−
Leucomalachite Green	+	+	+	−	−
Phenolphthalein	+	−	−	−	−

Key to blood solution concentrations:

A = 1:200
B = 1:2000
C = 1:20,000
D = 1:200,000
E = 1:400,000

Source: Ana Castelló Ponce and Fernando A. Verdú Pascual, (1999). "Critical Revision of Presumptive Tests for Bloodstains," *Forensic Science Communications,* Vol. 1, No. 2.

Blood

Blood screening methods are widely used by all laboratories and some crime scene units to exclude items in order to increase the efficiency of the DNA laboratory. *Leucomalachite green* is a color change reagent oxidized by peroxide that yields a colored reaction product (see table 12.1). The iron in blood hemoglobin catalyzes the color change. Strong oxidizers and other iron-containing compounds can result in false positives using these techniques. Proper personal protective equipment must be used while conducting these very sensitive and reactive chemicals. The screening tests may also consume the entire sample, leaving none for DNA analyses. The scientist must evaluate the benefits of the screening process to decide if screening may be an unnecessary risk to subsequent DNA analyses.

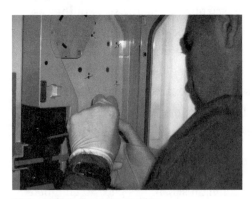
DNA analysis instrumentation

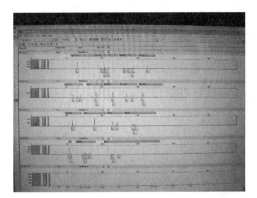

DNA data interpretation

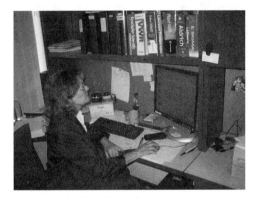

DNA technical leader reviewing casework data

Human blood screening methods are also used to identify bloodstains or liquids that may have the potential source attribute of human blood. Immunochromatographic test devices used in the medical community to detect human hemoglobin are now widely used in forensic laboratories to screen for human blood prior to DNA analysis. The OneStep ABAcard® HemaTrace® test device provided by Abacus Diagnostics is used for human blood screening tests. Interestingly, these tests can also test positive for the blood of other primates, such as chimpanzees, and for mustelids, such as ferrets, skunks, and weasels.

Seminal Fluid and Sperm

The prosecution of sexual offense cases relies heavily on the confirmed presence of seminal fluid and semen. A DNA profile can be developed from many other human tissues and fluids; however, the defense can claim that the resulting DNA profile was from a source other than seminal fluid or semen, and not the result of sexual assault.

Forensic nuclear DNA profile analysis does not identify the source of the human tissue. There are several methods used to collect and screen for the presence of seminal fluid and semen. There is also a variety of plant and animal tissues that can lead to a positive test result using these screening methods. A negative or exclusionary result usually means that no seminal fluid is present. However, with enough material, it may be possible to develop a DNA profile using the extremely sensitive DNA polymerase chain reaction short tandem repeat (PCR-STR) methods. Table 12.2 presents some of the procedures that are used.

Sexual Assault Evidence Kits

Historically, emergency room personnel have used collection items that were readily available, such as swabs and blood tubes, to collect evidence for sexual assault investigation. The victim's clothing and control samples

TABLE 12.2 *Methods Used to Collect and Screen for Presence of Seminal Fluid and Semen*

Visual examination of stain
- Dried, coarse, and crusted materials
- Noticeable stains on clothing, bedding, and other substrates
- Alternate light source creating fluorescence of stain or substrate

Sample collection
- Cuttings from clothing or other fabrics
- Swabs from surface of nonporous materials
- Patting the surface of stains with moistened filter paper or swabs
- Lifting small amounts of material from large stains

Brentamine
- Color test for seminal fluid

Prostate specific antigen (PSA)
- Visualization of PSA/antibody interface

Acid phosphatase
- Color test for seminal fluid

Microscopic visualization of sperm

of blood are placed in large bags or boxes and submitted to the forensic laboratory for analysis. Forensic laboratories have standardized the process by developing collection kits specifically for sexual assault evidence. The kit contains all collection tools, seals, and containers needed for blood, secretions, and trace evidence. Control blood tubes are also included for both the suspect and victim. Training programs have also been developed for emergency room personnel; this speacialization is entitled sexual assault nurse examiner (SANE).

Chemical screening and microscopic tests are applied to the items of evidence submitted in the sexual assault evidence kit. The kit is also used during an autopsy in a homicide investigation. The following basic evidence is collected:

- Control blood from suspect
- Vaginal, oral, and rectal swabs
- Vaginal, oral, and rectal smears on slides

- Dried secretion swabs
- Pubic hair controls
- Fingernail clippings
- Trace evidence (fibers and other debris)

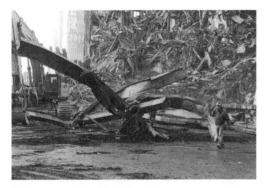

DNA was used to identify victims of the WTC disaster

DNA

The DNA laboratory receives all screened items that have tested positive for sperm, seminal fluid, blood, or other contact items, and controls that may contain DNA pertinent to a criminal case. The DNA must first be extracted from the nucleus of the cell, quantified, amplified, and then analyzed to develop a 13 loci short tandem repeat DNA profile. The 13 loci were identified and validated by the FBI and local laboratories. These loci were chosen due to no known phenotypic or metabolic alleles and the combined discriminating power of all 13 loci. Convicted offender and unknown forensic profiles are used to populate the Combined DNA Index System (CODIS), discussed in more detail in chapter 17.

There are three main extraction methods used in forensic DNA laboratories: Chelex®, organic, and differential. The Chelex extraction method uses a resin that consists of styrene divinylbenzene copolymers, which are added directly to the blood, bloodstain, or semen sample. The method relies upon the ability of the Chelex to prevent degradation of the DNA by inactivating nucleases that would potentially degrade the DNA. Procedures utilizing Chelex 100 chelating resin have been developed for

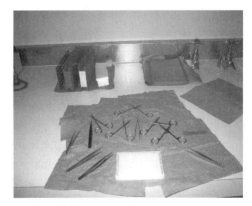

Sanitized laboratory tools

extracting DNA from forensic-type samples for use with the PCR that replace exposures to phenol extraction methods. Chelex procedures are simple, involve no organic solvents, and require fewer transfers. PCR inhibitors from substrate materials decrease amplification products when blood DNA is extracted from dirty samples.

The organic extraction procedure uses sodium dodecylsulfate (SDS) and proteinase K to open the nucleus of the cell and release the chromosomal DNA. A mixture of phenol and chloroform is used to separate the DNA from the remaining cellular debris. The organic procedure is time consuming and needs to be performed under a fume hood. The procedure also consists of multiple steps that can invite contamination. All reagents must also be disposed of according to laboratory safety policies. The organic method is used less frequently in laboratories to avoid exposure in handling phenol and chloroform.

Differential extraction is used to separate sperm from the female fraction of the evidence sample, usually found in the swabs collected in a sexual assault evidence kit. This method takes advantage of the fact the sperm heads are more resistant to the extraction process than the female epithelial cells found within the swabs. A typical evidence swab can contain blood, semen, seminal fluid, epithelial cells, saliva, hair, and a variety of contaminants. The semen must be separated from the female portion of the sample and compared to the suspect's DNA. Sodium dodecylsulfate (SDS), ethylenediamine tetraacetic acid (EDTA), and proteinase K are added to the evidence cell suspension, incubated at 37 degrees centigrade, and then centrifuged to form a sperm pellet. The lysed cells in the supernatant are removed for the female epithelial fraction of the sample. A mixture of SDS, EDTA, proteinase K, and dithiothreitol (DTT) mixture, lyses the remaining sperm heads. DNA quantitation is required to confirm that the required DNA is human and in a quantity sufficient to yield an acceptable profile with the DNA polymerase chain reaction (PCR). Too much DNA can cause off-scale measurements of DNA peaks. Too little DNA can lead to allele dropout because the DNA fails to amplify properly. The PCR reaction may fail due to inhibitors in the substrate, contaminants,

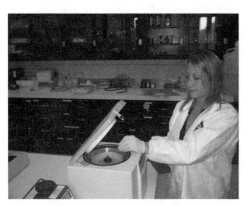

Scientist operating centrifuge

degraded DNA, insufficient quantity, or all of these factors. Real-Time PCR, RT-PCR®, is a new technique from Applied Biosystems that performs quantitation and amplification at the same time, increasing the efficiency of the process.

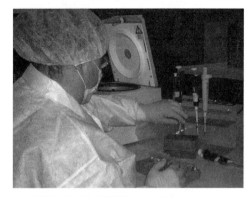

Scientist pipetting DNA extracts

The PCR reaction is responsible for the breakthrough in DNA procedures in which small amounts of DNA can be duplicated many times to manufacture or copy a great deal of DNA from small or invisible amounts of material. This technique duplicates all DNA molecules for approximately 30 cycles in a precise thermal cyclical sequence. The 30 cycles can yield approximately one billion copies of the targeted DNA or a product called an amplicon. The amplicon is used to develop a DNA profile from the original invisible amount of cellular material.

As described earlier, 13 of these unique short tandem repeats (STR) regions have been identified for use by the FBI as standardized forensic methods in the forensic community. The probability of a random match of one individual to all 13 STR regions is rarer than one in a trillion. Since the population of the world is approximately six billion, many forensic scientists state that the rarity of a profile containing all 13 STR regions is a categorical match or identity.

Frequently Asked Questions

Q: *What is the major impact of DNA technology?*

A: DNA technology provides a second tool (the first is fingerprints) that can place an individual at the crime scene. DNA technology is especially useful for violent crimes and sexual assaults, which generate blood, semen, and tissue transfer evidence.

Q: *What types of DNA processes are used in forensic casework?*

A: Mitochondrial DNA, Y STRs, and other STR loci are currently used in DNA casework and research. Y STR's are new short tandem repeats on the Y chromosome. RNA represents potential forensic tools of the future to provide tissue specificity and age of the source tissue.

Q: *How do labs address resulting case backlogs given the success of DNA technology?*

A: High performance teams, robotics, and miniaturization decrease cycle times and will increase the quality of the DNA laboratories in the future.

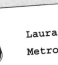

Laura Lake Residence
Metroland, New York

Forensic scientist Sara Herbst is newly assigned to the DNA casework section of the laboratory. Sara has just completed her DNA training, competency testing, mock trial exercise, and her cosigned 50 cases with a senior forensic scientist. The Laura Lake homicide is the first major case she has been assigned to work without direct supervision. She is determined to do the best job possible and identify any possible trace amounts of DNA that will help solve the case. The detection of blood from the victim upon any of the surfaces within the suspect's vehicle or clothing would place him at the scene of the crime.

Sara works with a team of technicians for over four weeks straight, including holidays and weekends, analyzing over 100 items of evidence. She finds no blood from the victim on any of the suspect's clothing, or stains found in his vehicle. She knows the suspect had cut himself on his hand when allegedly working as a landscaper. Sara and her team of technicians have thoroughly examined all items of evidence trying to identify a transfer of victim's blood to the suspect, with negative results. She *does* find the suspect's blood on top of his shoes. His alibi seemed to hold that he cut his hand while landscaping and the blood dripped on his shoes. She produces her final report for the case triage team and district attorney, realizing there was no information that would include or exclude the suspect.

CRIME SCENE

CHAPTER 13

Examining Firearms and Tool Marks

Firearms

Firearms are used in many violent crimes. Local and federal agencies, such as the Bureau of Alcohol, Tobacco, Firearms and Explosives (ATF) and the Federal Bureau of Investigation (FBI), dedicate significant resources to firearm technology and expertise. Most firearms examiners are sworn police officers who undergo intensive firearm operation and safety training at the police academy. Training includes coverage of federal and local laws and the associated criteria for enforcement of the law. For example, weapons such as machine guns are illegal to possess under any circumstance. Other weapons require a permit to carry or conceal. Some weapons can only be used for sport and hunting. The firearms examiner must understand these and other important distinctions in the law.

Police officers can possess and transport any type of firearm as part of their official duties. Transporting firearm evidence from the crime scene to the laboratory or to the courtroom is an essential part of their job responsibilities. Large police departments also require transport of firearms between laboratories, precincts, and various storage locations.

The organizational culture of police agencies often presents barriers that exclude civilian personnel from working in firearms. However, some departments have begun to integrate civilian personnel with sworn police in the firearms section. Civilians can be trained to serve as excellent firearms examiners.

Becoming a firearms examiner is one of the lengthiest apprenticeships in the forensic sciences. Training takes place almost exclusively with a mentor. There are very few, if any, complete academic training programs for forensic firearms examiners. Supplemental training programs have been developed by working groups within the forensic community and professional firearm organizations, such as the Association of Firearm and Tool Mark Examiners (AFTE). Essential components for firearm curricula include

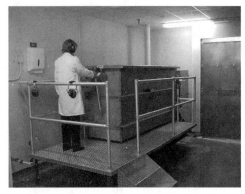

Firearms are test-fired into water tanks.

safety, a thorough reference collection of weapons and ammunition, a large volume and variety of weapons submitted to the laboratory for analysis, experienced training mentors, and a laboratory equipped and designed for the operation and examination of weapons.

Safety

The firearms unit routinely collects, handles, and examines firearms and ammunition. The most important consideration for every member of the unit, including supervisors, is safety. Many weapons involved in criminal investigations are of poor quality and are unsafe in any condition. Seemingly "safe" weapons have discharged, seriously injuring firearms examiners. Accidents are infrequent, but one accident in the firearms laboratory is too many.

Exposure to lead is also a safety concern. The firing range must have proper ventilation to remove lead vapors and particles from the air. The range must be cleaned to remove all traces of lead from the ceilings, walls, floor, and backstop. Firearms examiners undergo regular physical examinations that include blood tests to measure exposure to lead. The firearms examiner must be vigilant to protect against unsafe weapons and lead exposure with use of personal protective equipment.

Firearms Job Responsibilities and Tasks

The main tasks of firearms examiners include identification and operability of firearms and ammunition, ballistic comparison, distance determination, serial number restoration, identification of trace evidence deposited on firearms, and analysis of tool marks. Firearms and ammunition identification and operability are among the first skills learned by the firearms examiner. The weapon is inspected to ensure that it is safe and that no ammunition is in the chamber, magazine, or cylinder. Evidence receiving works closely with firearms examiners to inspect weapons for safety and trace evidence at the time they are submitted to the laboratory. Trace evidence, such as fingerprints and blood, may still be on the firearm. This trace evidence is essential to the prosecution of criminal cases. The firearms examiner also determines the make and model of the firearm and operability as per the penal code. Weapons are seized from suspects due to violations of the penal code, voluntarily surrendered, or are found property. The weapon must be defined and associated with the proper charge in the penal code.

The firearms examiner learns the nomenclature and firing mechanism of a weapon. This involves examining the weapon for any unsafe characteristics that may present a danger to the examiner, or to explain an accidental firing in a criminal case. Unsafe conditions typically found when examining weapons include the following:

- Dirty action
- Broken sear
- Bulged barrel
- Improperly replaced or missing parts
- Broken parts
- Defective safety
- Hairline cracks
- Overloads in ammunition
- Incorrect powder type
- Lodged ammunition in chamber

Next, the firearms examiner must properly describe and identify the weapon. Weapons can be classified into basic types such as shotguns, handguns (pistols and revolvers), automatics, semiautomatics, and single shots. The weapon is then further defined by make, model, and serial number and described in detail using standardized firearm nomenclature:

- Magazine
- Receiver
- Ejection port
- Ramp

The New York State Penal Code Section 265:
Firearms and Other Dangerous Weapons

Definitions. As used in this article and in article four hundred, the following terms shall mean and include:

1. "Machine gun" means a weapon of any description, irrespective of size, by whatever name known, loaded or unloaded, from which a number of shots or bullets may be rapidly or automatically discharged from a magazine with one continuous pull of the trigger and includes a sub-machine gun.

2. "Firearm silencer" means any instrument, attachment, weapon or appliance for causing the firing of any gun, revolver, pistol or other firearms to be silent, or intended to lessen or muffle the noise of the firing of any gun, revolver, pistol or other firearms.

3. "Firearm" means (a) any pistol or revolver; or (b) a shotgun having one or more barrels less than eighteen inches in length; or (c) a rifle having one or more barrels less than sixteen inches in length; or (d) any weapon made from a shotgun or rifle whether by alteration, modification, or otherwise if such weapon as altered, modified, or otherwise

- Barrel
- Lands and grooves
- Rifling
- Firing pin
- Extractor
- Bolt face
- Bolt
- Grips
- Frame
- Trigger
- Breech face
- Breech block

Ballistic comparisons are done with a comparison microscope that mounts a known (K) and questioned (Q) bullet or cartridge on the microscope for simultaneous side-by-side viewing of both items. The has an overall length of less than twenty-six inches; or (e) an assault weapon. For the purpose of this subdivision the length of the barrel on a shotgun or rifle shall be determined by measuring the distance between the muzzle and the face of the bolt, breech or breech lock when closed and when the shotgun or rifle is cocked; the overall length of a weapon made from a shotgun or rifle is the distance between the extreme ends of the weapon measured along a line parallel to the center line of the bore. Firearm does not include an antique firearm.

265.09 Criminal use of a firearm in the first degree.

1. A person is guilty of criminal use of a firearm in the first degree when he commits any class B violent felony offense as defined in paragraph (a) of subdivision one of section 70.02 and he either:

   (a) possesses a deadly weapon, if the weapon is a loaded weapon from which a shot, readily capable of producing death or other serious injury may be discharged; or

   (b) displays what appears to be a pistol, revolver, rifle, shotgun, machine gun or other firearm.

Criminal use of a firearm in the first degree is a class B felony.

rifling in the barrel of a weapon creates class characteristics of the weapon, such as six lands and grooves, that are twisted to the right. The machine tool that creates the rifling within the barrel leaves microscopic striations on the inside of the lands. These striations are imprinted upon the bullet. Test-fired bullets or other unknown bullets can be compared using the comparison microscope. An experienced firearms examiner develops an opinion as to whether the bullet was fired through a specific rifle barrel.

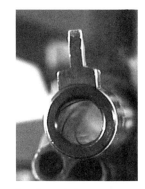

Lands and grooves within barrel of gun

Cartridges also develop unique microscopic images. The cartridge is pressed upon the breech face of the weapon upon firing. The tool used to finish the face of the breech also leaves microscopic markings that are imprinted on the rear of the cartridge upon firing. The firing pin leaves a unique mark upon the primer. There may also be unique

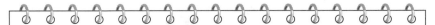

New technology has dramatically increased microscopic matching of bullets and cartridges to weapons. The Bureau of Alcohol, Tobacco, Firearms and Explosives (ATF) has created a database of digital ballistic images from bullets and cartridges fired from known weapons. This database is known as the National Integrated Ballistic Information Network (NIBIN). Cartridges and bullets are collected from crime scenes, digitized, and compared to the database of known (K) and questioned (Q) images. As recently as 10 years ago, these comparisons were only performed on a case-by-case basis. The technology is particularly effective in large metropolitan police departments that investigate gang-related and drive-by shootings.

markings placed on the sides of the cartridge by the extractor. The markings from the breech face, firing pin, and extractor are all used to compare test fires from a known weapon to questioned bullets or cartridges. The firearms examiner uses these comparisons to develop an opinion as to the source weapon of questioned bullets and cartridges.

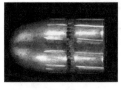

Land and groove impressions on projectile

A new challenge is how to best document microscopic observations. National accreditation guidelines from the American Society of Crime Laboratory Directors/Laboratory Accreditation Board state that documentation of observations must be made at the time of the observation. Verification of these observations is now performed using peer examiners. Traditionally, observations were performed with diagrams and Polaroid photography. Digital photography and computer controlled microscope stages are now used in the forensic laboratory to archive the specific location of these probative markings on the cartridge cases and bullets.

Tool Marks

Tool marks are commonly found in lesser offense cases, such as burglaries and larcenies. A tool may be used to break and enter a vehicle, residence, or a container with valuables. The variety of tools used is endless, from lock picks to large power saws and hammers. Firearms examiners are usually cross-trained in tool marks. Tool mark examination may be performed in the trace or microscopy section of the laboratory. Interestingly, some forensic scientists refer to firearm examination as "tool marks in the round." Training for tool mark examination begins with a review of the following common classes of tools:

- Filing
- Abrasive machining
- Boring
- Reaming
- Milling
- Turning
- Drilling
- Shaping
- Planing
- Sawing
- Prying

The definition of tool actions includes the following: fracturing, pinching, shearing, slicing, impressions, and scraping. Trainees practice making marks with a variety of tools, simulating the many uses and resulting patterns from tool cutting or abrasive actions.

Tools are often designed and manufactured with materials that cut and form softer compounds and natural materials, such as wood. The tool possesses class characteristics, for example, the shape of a pry bar. There are microscopic abrasions formed in the manufacturing process or by previous use. These class characteristics and microscopic imperfections are often left on the surface of the compromised item.

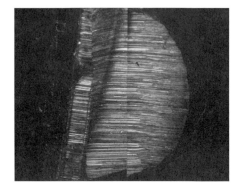

Trace evidence transfer between the tool, the suspect, and a broken or compromised item is often more important than the tool itself. For example, there may be fingerprints

Ballistic comparisons

or trace amounts of the suspect's perspiration on the handle of the tool. In this case, the handle is protected and submitted to fingerprint and DNA analysis. Paint can also transfer from the tool to the broken object or from the object to the tool. These types of trace evidence are included in the analysis at the lab.

Frequently Asked Questions

Q: *Where can an individual become trained as a firearms examiner and how long does it take?*

A: All firearm training is mentor based within the police forensic laboratory. Training can take several years, depending on the caseload and responsibilities of the mentor. There are armorer schools and training in the military that are directly related and applicable to forensic ballistics.

Q: *Do you need firearm experience to be a firearms examiner?*

A: No. Essential prerequisites for firearms examiners are hard work and interest (motivation).

CHAPTER 14

Toxicology, Hair, and Fibers

Toxicology

The toxicology section of the laboratory analyzes human biological tissues and fluids for poisons, prescription medications, and controlled substances. Criminal cases in toxicology typically relate to the impairment of psychomotor abilities as the cause of death.

Criminal cases related to impairment primarily involve motor vehicle accidents and investigations. Police officers observe erratic driving behavior and use standard police procedures to stop the driver. Through observations and physical agility tests, the police determine that the driver's ability to operate the vehicle is impaired. A breath screening device may be used to identify the presence of alcohol and to estimate the amount in the blood. The police officer requests the driver submit to a Breathalyzer test. This test may be insufficient to identify impairment by drugs. More sensitive blood or urine drug tests are required for investigations. Samples of blood and urine are obtained from the defendant through a court order. These samples are submitted to the forensic toxicology laboratory for analysis.

The medical examiner submits a postmortem tissue sample to the toxicology laboratory when the cause of death cannot be determined. In questionable death cases, the medical examiner has already ruled out natural or accidental causes of death. Toxicology analysis is performed for drugs, poisons, alcohol, and gases. The toxicology laboratory examines samples from the liver, brain, kidney, bile, vitreous humor, blood,

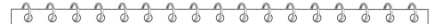

MARK'S STORY

"Boss, do you have a minute?" A serial murder investigation demonstrates how a case can be solved by an experienced forensic scientist with good old-fashioned memory. Toxicology evidence had been submitted to our lab in a questionable death case involving a child. The medical examiner could not be definitive on cause of death. Tissue samples had been obtained at the autopsy. A newly trained forensic toxicologist performed routine screens for poisons, gases, controlled substances, and prescription medications, all with negative results.

Larry had 30 years experience as a forensic scientist and several advanced degrees in toxicology. Larry practically lived in the lab; his nights and weekends were spent working on cases and experimenting with new methods. Occasionally, Larry poked his head in my door to say, "Boss, do you have a minute?" When that happened, I knew to stop whatever I was doing, send everyone out of the office except for Larry, and shut the door. When Larry politely asked if I "had a minute," he was on the verge of solving a big case.

In the triage team meeting to discuss the case, Larry had thought that the unusual family name sounded familiar. He had spent all weekend searching through old records and logbooks of laboratory submissions from previous cases. Sure enough, Larry found that another child had died suspiciously in the same family more than 10 years before. A subsequent criminal investigation led to the arrest and conviction of the child's uncle. The case was re-opened due to the encyclopedic memory of the senior scientist.

urine, stomach contents, and hair to identify and quantify any substance that may cause death.

Appropriate samples are obtained at autopsy. Toxicology analysis proceeds in a logical sequence to identify and quantify controlled substances, poisons, and alcohol. Two differences between the drug and toxicology departments are the sample matrix and detection levels used. The drug section analyzes pills, tablets, powders, and liquids that may be pure or contaminated with impurities. The toxicology section analyzes body tissues and fluids for very small amounts of pure drugs or associated metabolites. These compounds can be in very low concentrations (ng/ml or µg/ml) and difficult to detect and quantify. The medical examiner and crime scene team must be diligent in preventing contamination from known control samples or stomach contents during the autopsy.

Scientific literature and medical experts are consulted in order to compare level of impairment or lethal dosage to the observed amounts of drugs in the tissue or fluid collected from the autopsy. The amount of pure drug in the system and level of impairment depend upon the victim's metabolism, size, time of impairment or death versus time of ingestion, and any contrary effects from multiple drugs or alcohol. Common techniques used in a toxicology laboratory consist of immunoassay screenings for drugs of abuse, such as the following:

- Methamphetamine
- Amphetamines
- Barbiturates
- Benzodiazepines
- Cannabinoids
- Cocaine metabolites
- Methadone
- Opiates
- Phencylidine
- Trycyclic antidepressants
- Acetaminophin
- Phenytoin
- Salicylates

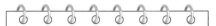

Table 14.1 is an example of how sensitive toxicology techniques can detect very small amounts of compounds that cause impairment in GHB, the "date-rape" drug.

The molecular confirmation of drugs identified in the screening process using gas chromatograph mass spectrometers are always compared to a standard mass spectra derived from appropriate pure controls.

Hair

The analysis and comparison of hair in the laboratory is now used primarily as a screening process for DNA analysis. For many years, the microscopic evaluation and comparison of hair was routinely performed in forensic laboratories using comparison microscopes. Microscopic comparison of hairs is a tedious process requiring weeks or months for a single investigation.

TABLE 14.1 *Summary of Therapeutic, Toxic, and Postmortem Laboratory Findings Following Exposure to Gamma-Hydroxybutyric Acid (GHB) and Related Compounds (Hornfeldt, Lothridge, & Downs, 2002)*

THERAPEUTIC DRUG CONCENTRATIONS						
Ingested Substance	Ingested Dose	Measured Substance(s)	Source(s)	Concentration**		Reference
GHB	3 g repeated after 4 hrs (26.4–52.4 mg/kg)	GHB	Plasma	Two doses resulted in two peaks. Means = 62.8 mg/L (SD=27.4) and 91.2 mg/L (SD=25.6), N=6		Scharf et al. 1998B
GHB	25 mg/kg	GHB	Plasma	55 mg/L (range 24-88 mg/L)		Ferrara et al. 1993
	50 mg/kg	GHB	Plasma	90 mg/L (range 51-158 mg/L)		
GHB	25 mg/kg	GHB	Plasma	Mean = 54 mg/L (SD=19), N=10		Ferrara et al. 1992
TOXIC DRUG CONCENTRATIONS						
Ingested Substance	Ingested Dose	Measured Substance(s)	Source(s)	Concentration	Comments	Reference
1,4-BD	6.3–8.4 g	1,4-BD	Urine	Undetectable	GCS=3*	Zvosec et al. 2001
		GHB	Urine	415 mg/L		
1,4-BD	4.5 g	1,4-BD	Urine	Undetectable	GCS=II*; labile level of conciousness	Zvosec et al. 2001
		GHB	Serum	317 mg/L		
		GHB	Urine	716 mg/L		
1,4-BD	Unknown	1,4-BD	Urine	Undetectable	Withdrawal; same patient as above, subsequent event	Zvosec et al. 2001
		GHB	Urine	5,140 mg/L		
GHB	Unknown	GHB	Serum	125 mg/L	Ethanol, a coingestant; GCS=6*	Louagie et al. 1997
GHB	Unknown	GHB	Serum	101 mg/L	1HR post-ingestion; GCS=3*; 2-month delay in analysis	Dyer et al. 1994
		GHB	Urine	141,000 mg/L		
GHB	Unknown	GHB	Serum	0 mg/L	1HR post-ingestion; GCS=3*; 2-month delay in analysis	Dyer et al. 1994
		GHB	Urine	1,857 mg/L		
GHB	Unknown	GHB	Serum	0 mg/L	1HR post-ingestion; GCS=3*; 2-month delay in analysis	Dyer et al. 1994
		GHB	Urine	521 mg/L		
GHB	Unknown	GHB	Urine	1,975 mg/L	THC metabolite also present; severe ataxia	Stephens and Baselt 1994
POSTMORTEM DRUG CONCENTRATIONS						
Ingested Substance	Ingested Dose	Measured Substance(s)	Source(s)	Concentration	Comments	Reference
1,4-BD	26 g (estimated to be 320 mg/kg)	1,4-BD	Heart Blood	78 mg/L		Martin and Duer 2001
			Urine	870 mg/L		
		GHB	Heart Blood	416 mg/L		
			Urine	1810 mg/L		

TABLE 14.1 *Summary of Therapeutic, Toxic, and Postmortem Laboratory Findings Following Exposure to Gamma-Hydroxybutyric Acid (GHB) and Related Compounds (continued)*

Ingested Substance	Ingested Dose	Measured Substance(s)	Source(s)	Concentration	Comments	Reference
1,4-BD	5.4–10.8 g (estimated to be 95-n-189 mg/kg)	1,4-BD	Blood	220 mg/L		Zvosec et al. 2001
			Urine	1756 mg/L		
		GHB	Blood	837 mg/L		
			Urine	1161 mg/L		
1,4-BD	20 g (estimated to be 300 mg/kg)	1,4-BD	Urine	845 mg/L		McCutcheon et al. 2000
		GHB	Blood	432 mg/L		
			Urine	5430 mg/L		
1,4-BD	Unknown	1,4-BD	Blood	7.6 mg/L		Kraner et al. 2000
			Urine	146 mg/L		
			Bile	0 mg/L		
			Vitreous H.	12.3 mg/L		
		GHB	Blood	280 mg/L		
			Urine	6,171 mg/L		
			Bile	218 mg/L		
			Vitreous H.	324 mg/L		
GHB	Unknown	GHB	Blood	140 mcg/g	ethanol, fenfluramine, & norfenfluramine also present	Timby et al. 2000
			Urine	620 mcg/g		
GHB	Unknown	GHB	Blood	170 mcg/g	ethanol & nordazepam also present	Timby et al. 2000
			Urine	300 mcg/g		
GHB	Unknown	GHB	Heart Blood	66 mg/L	second case may have also involved ingestion of gamma-butyrolactone	Marinetti et al. 2000
			Urine	1260 mg/L		
GHB	Unknown	GHB	Heart Blood	15 mg/L		
			Urine	150 mg/L		
GHB	Unknown	GHB	Blood	11.5 mg/L	heroin was a co-ingestant: morphine and 6-monoacetyl-morphine also present	Ferrara et al. 1995
			Urine	258.3 mg/L		
			Bile	57.0 mg/L		
			Vitreous H.	84.3 mg/L		
NONE	Unknown	GHB	Blood, N=20	0-168 mg/L	mean 25 mg/L	Fieler et al. 1998
			Urine, N=8	0 mg/L		
NONE	Unknown	GHB	Blood, N=13	0-197 mg/L	mean 57 mg/L	Elliot 2001
			Urine, N=13	0-217 mg/L	mean 56 mg/L	

* Glascow Coma Scale
** Those laboratory values reported as mg/mL converted to mg/L for consistency.
Source: Hornfeldt, Lothridge, & Downs, 2002

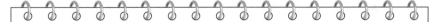

MARK'S STORY

An interesting case involved a woman who died in her sleep. The medical examiner could not find any medical explanation for the cause of death. All normal tissues and fluids were submitted to the laboratory for routine toxicology analysis. The police department was suspicious because the woman was in good health and had no unusual family medical history. There were reports that the husband and wife had quarreled, but not to the extent to which foul play was suspected.

I asked a toxicologist to perform all possible analyses and to rerun tests for heavy metals or halogen containing poisons. One week later, the toxicologist came to my office and said, "Boss, I have something on that questionable death: chloroform." I asked that he repeat the analysis and have a peer—another scientist—repeat the work for confirmation. Results confirmed the original conclusion and we notified the police agency. Confronted with the results, the husband confessed to applying a chloroform-soaked rag to his wife's face while she was sleeping so he could steal her rings.

The husband was convicted of manslaughter and sentenced to 20 years in the state penitentiary. This was an unusual case that was solved by a persistent scientist who would not give up until all available science and technology were applied to the case.

The results of microscopic comparisons depend on characteristics of known controls submitted along with the questioned samples. Microscopic analysis of hair evaluates questioned (Q) hairs for the suitability of molecular comparison between known DNA (K) from the suspect or victim. Microscopic analysis can determine the class characteristics of hair and confirm the presence of a root. Some laboratories have added this function to the serologist or DNA scientist and created a new job description, known as bio-trace analyst.

The combination of DNA analysis and microscopy has added efficiency to the evidence screening process. This is a significant change in the forensic laboratory. It is driven by the increased definitive power and sensitivity of DNA technology. It is now possible to obtain a nuclear DNA profile from a hair root and a mitochondrial DNA profile from the hair shaft. The results of these analyses can be categorically negative and exclude an individual as the source for the hair. An exclusionary mitochondrial DNA result can be more important in a criminal case than inclusion. The ability to determine that a hair (Q) is definitively not associated with the (K) suspect, victim, or other individuals present at the scene, adds probative information and great efficiency to criminal investigation.

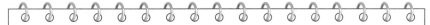

Imagine taking a full vacuum-cleaner bag and spreading its contents out on a large table for analysis. That is exactly what forensic scientists do. First, the examiner separates the debris into general categories suitable for microscopic analysis. Using a stereo microscope, the examiner separates human hairs from fibers and other debris. This is followed by microscopic comparisons using comparison microscopes. The process is also used prior to other analyses in the laboratory to prevent loss or contamination of trace evidence. DNA technology has started to replace much of the microscopic comparison of human hairs.

The analysis of a hair found upon the body of a homicide victim is compared to the DNA of the victim and suspect. The hair examiner first determines if the hair is human, animal, fiber, or debris. If the hair is human, the body area (e.g., head, body, pubic, limb) and race (e.g, Caucasian, Mongoloid, Negroid) can be identified. Other characteristics of hair include damage, forced removal, external hair dye, and bleaching treatments.

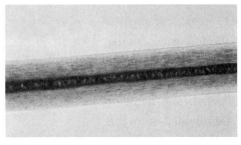

Microscopic view of hair

If the hair is human and contains a root, the evidence is packaged and forwarded to the DNA section for analysis. Nuclear DNA is used to analyze a hair root and mitochondrial DNA is used for a hair shaft. When nuclear DNA is used to analyze the root of the hair, suspects can be included or excluded as the source of the hair. When mitochondrial DNA analysis is performed on a hair shaft, the statistical analysis is less definitive for inclusion. When mitochondrial DNA analysis results in exclusion, the results are certain.

Further analyses are also possible to identify nonhuman material. For example, animal hairs can be identified by species, such as dog, cat, deer, mouse, elk, or moose. Private laboratories perform animal hair DNA analysis. Hairs from pets can be found everywhere in the pet owner's home,

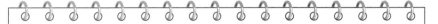

Wayne Williams Case

The Wayne Williams case is a good example of how DNA technology is being applied to cold cases involving hair comparison.

In November 2006, Williams's lawyers asked that they be allowed to run comparative DNA tests on dozens of animal hairs and two human hairs linking Williams to the slayings of 11 black men and boys in 1982. When Williams was tried, comparative human DNA testing had never been used in a criminal case, and the technology for testing animal DNA was not yet in existence. Although the Fulton County, Georgia district attorney decided in early 2007 not to oppose Williams's request to run the tests, the man believed to be Atlanta's notorious child killer still has significant hurdles to overcome in his 25-year-old quest for a new trial.

vehicle, and clothing. If a suspect was in the victim's residence or vehicle, there is a good chance of finding pet hair on the suspect.

Fibers

Fibers are a valuable source of trace evidence with potential to add much information to the criminal investigation. The significance of fiber evidence *increases* if other, more definitive types of evidence, such as fingerprints or DNA, are not conclusive. The first task for the forensic scientist is to classify all of the fibers found in the vacuumings submitted from a crime scene or collected from items of evidence. Fibers are divided into the categories shown in Table 14.2.

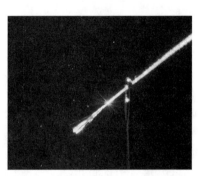

Fiber

The recognition and collection of the fibers is done by combing, vacuuming, scraping, taping, and picking. Combing is used to collect fibers from carpets, clothing, and hair. Scraping is done with a large spatula or similar object, directly over a collection table covered with clean butcher paper. The debris is packaged in envelopes and forwarded with the butcher paper to the microscopy section. The taping process uses two- to four-inch clear packing tape, pressed on the fabric or

TABLE 14.2 *Three Categories of Fibers*

1. Natural Fibers	2. Man-Made Fibers	3. Mineral Fibers
• Animal Fibers	• Acetate	• Glass
– Wool	• Acrylics	– Asbestos
– Other animal hairs	• Nylon	• Metal
Alpaca	• Glass	• Carbon
Camel	• Modacrylic	
Angora	• Aramid	
Cashmere	– Nomex, Kevlar	
Mohair	• Olefin	
– Silk	• Polyester	
	• Rayon	
• Vegetable	• Nylon	
– Seed hairs	• Rayon	
Cotton	• Saran	
Kapak	• Spandex	
– Bast fibers	• Triacetate	
Flax	• Vinyl	
Hemp	• Vinyon	
Jute		
Ramie		
– Leaf fibers		
Abaca		
Sisal		

clothing for trace evidence. Trace fiber or hair evidence adheres to the tape for later analysis. There are instruments specifically designed to analyze and identify fibers collected with adhesive tape. The Foster & Freeman FX5 Fibre Finder® scans for fibers that have been collected with clear adhesive tape and placed on 8.5 × 11 inch clear acetate sheets. Picking is simply done with a pair of sterile or disposable tweezers. Vacuuming is done with a specialized vacuum cleaner that is equipped with macro and micro filters placed within the vacuum hose to collect large and then the smallest of fibers.

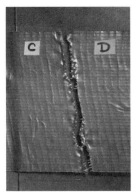

Matching fibers
in duct tape/front

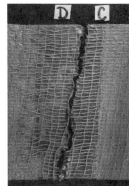

Matching fibers
in duct tape/back

Once collected, fibers can be identified and compared using microscopy, fluorescence, optical, Fourier transform infrared spectroscopy (FTIR), microspectrometry, or thin-layer chromatography properties. Microscopic properties include the following:

- Color
- Diameter
- Presence and quantity of deluster agents
- Texturizing agents
- Cross-sectional shape
- Surface characteristics

Fluorescent properties are exhibited by some fibers. Factors that influence the brightness and color of fluorescence include detergents, brighteners, bleaches, and other additives. Optical properties include the following:

- Interference colors—comparisons that use a polarizing microscope and position fibers in maximum brightness
- Pleochroism—comparisons that use a polarizing microscope with plain polarized light. Any change in color while rotating the fiber is called pleochroic; similar fibers exhibit the same pleochroic characteristics.

FTIR microspectrophotometry yields a spectra unique for the synthetic fiber. Infrared spectra of the known standard (K) are compared to the unknown forensic sample (Q). The microspectrophotometer is used to measure the color of the fiber. Multiple readings are taken from multiple fibers to obtain representative spectra for comparison purposes. Thin-layer chromatography is needed to compare the dyes used to color the fibers. A variety of extraction solvent reagents are used to select the best extraction technique.

Any differences noted when questioned fibers are compared to the known standard involves a categorical exclusion of the questioned fiber. For example, all characteristics of the questioned fiber and known standard may be identical except for the separation of dyes when subjected to a thin-layer chromatography separation technique. The differences in thin-layer results are enough to exclude the control as being the source of the questioned fiber. The recognition, collection, protection, identification, and comparison of fibers are tedious and exacting analyses that require significant patience and expertise. It can take one scientist weeks and months of analyses for a single homicide case.

Frequently Asked Questions

Q: *Do most laboratories have trained microscopists working with fiber comparisons?*

A: Resource limitations have resulted in fewer microscopy sections. The laboratory must target personnel and equipment toward the most productive types of evidence. Large city, state, and federal laboratories can justify a microscopy unit due to diverse caseloads with a large volume of cases.

Q: *How do scientists receive training and experience for microscopy and trace analysis work in a forensic laboratory?*

A: It is important for young scientists to develop mentor relationships in academic and forensic laboratories. Mentors should have extensive experience in forensic microscopy and be well known in the field. Professional organizations provide workshops with microscope vendors that provide opportunities to build mentor relationships. Some forensic academic programs include course work in microscopy.

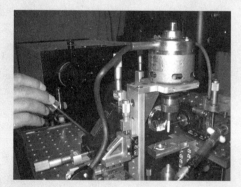

Fiber research

CHAPTER 15

The Case Triage Team
and Hypothesis Development

The basis for validation and exclusion of hypotheses is the scientific method. In criminal investigations, data is used to support (validate) or refute (exclude) a hypothesis. The scientific method includes processes of inductive and deductive reasoning. Data developed from scientific evidence, behavioral analysis, interviews, timelines, and new forensic technologies help to solve the criminal investigation. Ultimately a hypothesis leads to a lawful arrest, prosecution, conviction, or exclusion of a suspect.

During criminal investigations, information is gathered and used by the case triage team (CTT) to validate with a degree of certainty a theory of how the crime was committed. The CTT consists of experts from multiple agencies invested in the resolution of the crime, including detectives, supervisors, forensic scientists, and other specialists. Just as important as validating theories is the categorical

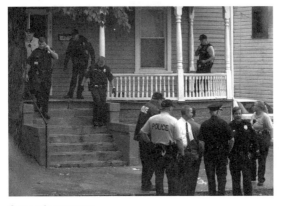

Case triage team

exclusion of theories of the crime and suspects. It is interesting to note that DNA technology is used to *exclude* more than one-third of suspects before arrest. Thus DNA is instrumental in helping to avoid wrongful arrests, wrongful convictions, and wrongful imprisonment.

The development of a hypothesis about the crime scene is critical in complex cases. It is often difficult to establish the sequence of events that transpired during the commission of a crime. Anything that cannot be explained during the investigation needs to be resolved. Otherwise the team risks an uncertain hypothesis. For example, there may be multiple DNA profiles, sets of fingerprints, hairs, fibers, and footprints developed from the evidence recovered at the scene. The unknown Qs may not match any known controls (Ks) from the victim, suspect, or individuals present at the crime scene. These unexplained items of evidence can weaken or even ultimately exclude a hypothesis.

The police department designates a senior detective to take charge of every homicide investigation. The detective in charge assimilates information developed by all personnel working on the case, including detectives, the medical examiner, and the laboratory. The detective in charge holds frequent meetings of the CTT. The detective develops hypotheses to explain how the crime occurred in order to identify possible suspects. These hypotheses and their associated facts will support the elements of the crime according to the penal code of the appropriate jurisdiction. Sources of the information used are limited only to the experience, contacts, resources, and time available to the detective.

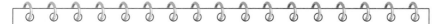

DNA Helps to Exclude Suspects

One-third of all suspects are excluded *prior to being arrested* when DNA evidence is available. Would these suspects have been excluded before DNA technology was available? It is difficult to say. An interesting research project would be to identify exclusions that result from the use of DNA technology, and recommend improvements to the investigative process. Cold cases are now investigated with intact DNA. The application of new technology to old casework has identified wrongful convictions and led to the release from prison of the wrongly convicted.

The *lead desk* applies techniques and principles from the scientific method to solve crimes. But if detectives were asked to explain the inductive and deductive reasoning process using the scientific method, they would respond with a blank stare. Detectives intuitively use these

The Lead Desk Concept

A homicide investigation at a secluded summer camp provides a good example of the lead desk. The command post was set up in a cottage adjacent to the homicide scene with permission of the owner. Fifteen seasoned investigators were assigned to the case. Dedicating a significant number of experienced detectives right at the beginning can help solve the case quickly.

The case involved an elderly woman who had enjoyed many summers at the lake with her husband. After he died and against the wishes of her family, the woman decided to spend one last summer at the camp by herself, and then put her home up for sale. But one quiet summer day a neighbor noticed that the door to her home was wide open. Checking, the neighbor found her lying dead in her kitchen, the victim of multiple stab wounds.

Investigators worked 24/7 knowing that their concerted effort could break the case. The team of 15 investigators at the command post represented an impressive $1 million in combined annual salaries. Every morning and every night, the team would report their progress to the lead desk—a seasoned investigator with over 30 years experience. Officers with much higher rank would defer to the lead on all issues related to the investigation. Command officers would ask what resources were needed—funding, personnel, equipment—and they would somehow make it happen.

The lead desk became the hub for every scrap of information related to the case. Evidence poured in, including statements, photos, timelines, warrants, and phone recordings. Witnesses and suspects were identified and statements taken. Warrants were obtained and additional leads were assigned. The lead desk approved all pending assignments and delegated new assignments.

Notably, the only technology used by the lead desk was a box of alphabetically sorted 3 × 5 index cards. The lead desk investigator became known as a "water cooled computer," police slang for the brains of the operation. The lead desk systematically eliminated all suspects until finally only one remained. (It is then said that this suspect *cannot be excluded.*)

Within three weeks, the lead desk detective presented the team's findings along with a hypothesis and the name of the potential suspect to the prosecutor. The prosecutor issued a warrant and the suspect was arrested for the homicide.

FIGURE 15.1 *Hypothesis Development*

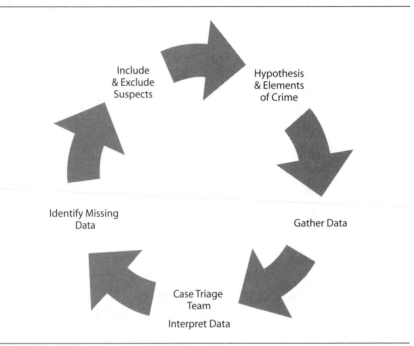

principles to solve the case. Data mining computer programs with intuitive algorithms have been developed to function as the lead desk; however, there is no substitute for an experienced detective managing the lead desk. Suspect behavior patterns, timelines, new forensic technologies, recidivism, serendipity—all are combined along with human reasoning to solve the case.

The Scientific Method

A basic flow chart and description of the scientific method in forensic science can be seen in Figure 15.1. Critical elements include the gathering and interpretation of data by the case triage team (CTT), the recognition that critical data is missing and needs to be sought, the inclusion and exclusion of suspects based on key information, and the identification of hypotheses to determine how the crime was committed.

Hypothesis Testing, Inductive and Deductive Reasoning

Seventeenth-century philosopher Francis Bacon believed that making a large number of observations could lead to grand theories that could explain nature. *Inductive reasoning* involves making specific observations that lead to general theories. Inductive reasoning begins with a set of observations. These lead to a generalization or the beginnings of a hypothesis or a "best guess." In a criminal case, observations include data from laboratory analyses, the behavior patterns of suspects and victims, timelines, interviews, and statements. All types of communication relevant to the investigation—including written, verbal, computer, email, and cell phones—represent observations.

Deductive reasoning moves from the general to the specific and was first described by French mathematician and philosopher, Rene Descartes. Descartes postulated that specific observations could be explained by thinking about general ideas or theories. Fictional detective Sherlock Holmes popularized the use of both inductive and deductive reasoning to solve crimes.

Deductive reasoning moves from general to specific. Deductive reasoning looks at all the characteristics of the offender, behavior patterns, prior convictions, and all physical evidence. Deductive reasoning would develop as follows:

Premise 1. The majority of sexual offenders are responsible for sexual offenses after they are released from prison.

Premise 2. The majority of sexual offenders return to their home area or the same geographical area after being released from prison.

Premise 3. The majority of sex offenders began their criminal career committing burglaries and other lesser offenses.

Premise 4. The DNA data bank authorizes the collection of DNA (buccal swab) from lesser offenses.

Hypothesis: It is likely that the sexual offender has contributed a DNA sample to the DNA data bank due to the conviction of a lesser offense, such as burglary.

Note the terms "majority" and "likely." Statistical probability can determine the likeliness or certainty of a convicted burglar having committed one or more sexual offenses. For example, in a specific geographical area, a detective could obtain data on the number and types of lesser offense incidents, convictions, and contributors to the DNA data bank. The resulting probability could be significant due to a high recidivism rate for burglary and sexual assaults. Probability and statistics are quite useful and sometimes the only way to analyze data in a given situation.

Errors or omissions in data and facts that are unknown weaken hypothesis formation. A certain number of convicted "lesser offenders" and "sexual offenders" *have not* contributed a sample to the DNA data bank. A certain number of sexual offenders have not committed lesser offenses. Some offenders do not return to the same neighborhood to commit the same crimes. However, the lead desk detective and crime scene team must work smart, focusing their finite resources on strategies that have a high probability of success, such as the known recidivists.

Inductive reasoning uses a series of observations as building blocks to form a premise or hypothesis. A hypothesis is a work in progress that may or may not be correct. Several hypotheses may be developed at the same time from the data streaming into the CTT. One hypothesis is eventually formed to explain the totality of all observations. Any observation, data, or fact that does not fit the hypothesis must be explained, eliminated, or result in a change of the hypothesis. The following is an example of how observations lead to a hypothesis in an inductive argument:

Premise 1. A sexual assault occurred in the Third Precinct.

Premise 2. Many sexual offenders have been convicted of burglaries in the Third Precinct.

Premise 3. Burglars have a high rate of recidivism.

Hypothesis: The sexual assault in the Third Precinct was most probably committed by an individual with a prior conviction for burglary.

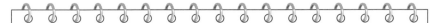

Preconceived Bias, Perception, and Inference

Disparities in perceptions or preconceived biases by participants might facilitate certain, and possibly wrong, inferences. Perception is the mental process by which people gather, organize, interpret, and evaluate information; each participant could perceive the same incident or conversation differently. In the interrogation setting, this not only includes differences in perceptions between the investigator and the suspect, but also between investigators.

Source: FBI Law Enforcement Bulletin, December 2006, Volume 75, Number 12.

Forensic scientists and detectives must keep an open mind from the beginning of the investigation, attempting to gather all possible data to support a hypothesis that explains the totality of events leading to the commission of the crime. This is the most difficult part of the investigative process. Detectives and forensic scientists instantly recall prior knowledge of similar crimes and correlate those factors to the new case. Experience is priceless when investigating criminal cases; however, forensic science relies on evidence that is factual and unbiased. Detectives seek advice from peers to review data with a "clear eye." Data derived from the analysis of evidence has no stake in the outcome of the investigation and provides a categorical exclusion or inclusion with varying degrees of uncertainty.

Gathering and Interpreting Data with the Case Triage Team

One of the most effective ways to analyze and interpret the data is to establish a case triage team (CTT). The CTT analyzes and interprets all data collected for the case, applies the data to the proper penal law charge, and recommends a hypothesis or fact pattern for the sequence of events leading to the commission of the crime. The CTT also consists of individuals who have the authority to redirect resources for the detective or laboratory to enable assignments to be completed in a timely manner. Multi-agency, multidisciplinary teams focused upon on specific cases increase the efficiency and quality of the investigation. Members of the CTT usually consist of the following:

- The prosecutor
- The medical examiner
- All forensic scientists performing analyses on the case
- Crime scene personnel
- The lead detective
- Other scientific and medical experts

What are the sources of data for the detective? Forensic evidence, statements, witnesses, and past behavior patterns from all individuals associated with the case are all primary sources of information for the detective. All evidence associated with the case will be sorted into known (K) and questioned (Q) data with information indicating the item number, forensic discipline, report date, and forensic scientist performing the analysis. An

FIGURE 15.2 *Evidence Analyses Progress Chart*

	Item #	LF	Ser	Nuclear DNA	Low Copy DNA	Mito DNA	FA	LP	Tox	Trace Hair Fiber Impressions	QD	Drugs	FS	R
Known Control														
Vic Control Blood	K1	CS												
Vic Control Prints	K2	CS												
Susp Control Blood	K1	CS												
Susp Control Prints	K4	CS												
Victim 10 Prints	K8	CS												
Suspect 10 Prints	K9	CS												
EMT Shoes	K10	CS												
Susp Shoes														
Autopsy														
Blood	K11	A												
Urine	K12	A												
Liver	K13	A												
Bile	K14	A												
Vitreous Humor	K15	A												
Stomach Contents	K16	A												
Prescription Drugs	K17	A												
Other Standards	K18..n	A												
Questioned														
Blood of Floor	Q1..n	CS												
Latent Prints	Q2..n	CS												
Shoe Prints	Q5..n	CS												
Blood on Bludgeon	Q6..n	CS												
Vehicle														
Latent Prints	Q7..n	V												
Blood	Q8..n	V												

LF = location found	SER = serology	CS = crime scene	A = autopsy	K = known	QD = questioned documents
Q = questioned	FA = firearms	LP - latent prints	V = victim	R = report	FS = forensic scientists

evidence chart (Figure 15.2) documents the progress of analyses in the lab and is an essential part of an investigation.

The left-hand column lists the description of all the known standards (K) and questioned (Q) items for analyses. The management of the evidence from a homicide case can be very complex when more than one laboratory (such as private and public) and multiple section analyses are involved. Human hairs with roots can be submitted to the public laboratory for nuclear DNA analyses and come back with negative results; that is, no nuclear DNA was found. The hair shafts may be subsequently submitted to a federal or private laboratory for mitochondrial DNA analyses. A multisection case could involve both blood and fingerprints

FIGURE 15.3 *Select Forensic Techniques and Materials*

Abrasives	Image analyses
Adhesives	Inks
Anthropology	Latent prints
Arson	Lubricants
Automobile	Metallurgy
Bank security dyes	Missing persons
Building materials	Paint
Bullet jacket alloys	Pepper spray
Caulks	Pharmaceuticals
Chemical unknown	Polymers
Computers	Product tampering
Controlled substances	Questioned documents
Cords	Racketeering records
Crime scene reconstruction	Ropes
Cryptanalysis	Safe insulation
Disaster squad	Sealants
DNA	Serial numbers
Electronic devices	Shoe prints
Explosives	Soils
Explosive residues	Tapes
Facial imaging	Tire treads
Feathers	Tool marks
Fibers	Toxicology
Firearms	Videos
Glass	Weapons of mass destruction
Gun shot residue	Woods
Hairs	

Source: FBI Evidence Handbook, 2003, Web: *209.85.165.104/search?q=cache: al1XGK1uUg4J:www.fbi.gov/hq/lab/handbook/forensics.pdf+fbi+handbook&hl=en&ct= clnk&cd=2&gl=us*

on a gun. Three types of analyses (DNA, fingerprints, and ballistics) must be performed on one item of evidence. Two important fields in the chart are the forensic scientist and report date. The detective is most concerned with the forensic scientist responsible for the analysis, her final laboratory report, and expert opinion.

There is no limit to the scientific disciplines used to gather data in formulating a hypothesis in forensic science. A detective must become very

New York State Penal Law Section 125.00.

Homicide defined. Homicide means conduct which causes the death of a person or an unborn child with which a female has been pregnant for more than twenty-four weeks under circumstances constituting murder, manslaughter in the first degree, manslaughter in the second degree, criminally negligent homicide, abortion in the first degree or self-abortion in the first degree.

§ 125.25 Murder in the second degree. A person is guilty of murder in the second degree when:

1. With intent to cause the death of another person, he causes the death of such person or of a third person; . . . or
2. Under circumstances evincing a depraved indifference to human life, he recklessly engages in conduct which creates a grave risk of death to another person, and thereby causes the death of another person; or
3. Acting either alone or with one or more other persons, he commits or attempts to commit robbery, burglary, kidnapping, arson, rape in the first degree, criminal sexual act in the first degree, sexual abuse in the first degree, aggravated sexual abuse, escape in the first degree, or escape in the second degree, and, in the course of and in further-

familiar with the scientists and the analyses they perform to formulate the best hypothesis from the best data. Some of these major disciplines of forensic science have been covered in previous chapters. All of the disciplines rely on comparison of known standards (Ks) to unknown evidence items (Qs). The types of comparisons or analyses of Ks and Qs are limited only by the techniques and instrumentation available in laboratories. Larger laboratories in the federal government, states, or municipalities offer a wider variety of chemical and instrumental analyses to compare on the molecular level most of the substances. The experienced investigator will know the capabilities of the laboratory for each one of the techniques listed in the Figure 15.3. An experienced crime scene technician and detectives will be aware of the laboratory limits of detection and sensitivity for all of types of analyses. The crime scene detective will then have a new set of eyes when processing a crime scene and formulating a hypothesis. There is a potential comparison of Ks and Qs for all of these substances and more. The detective must remember the Locard principle and always consider ance of such crime or of immediate flight therefrom, he, or another participant, if there be any, causes the death of first, second or third degree, sexual abuse in the first degree, aggravated sexual abuse in the first, second, third or fourth degree, or incest in the first, second or third degree, against a person less than fourteen years old, he or she intentionally causes the death of such person.

4. Under circumstances evincing a depraved indifference to human life, and being eighteen years old or more, the defendant recklessly engages in conduct which creates a grave risk of serious physical injury or death to another person less than eleven years old and thereby causes the death of such person; or

5. Being eighteen years old or more, while in the course of committing rape in the first, second or third degree, criminal sexual act in the first, second or third degree, sexual abuse in the first degree, aggravated sexual abuse in the first, second, third or fourth degree, or incest in the first, second or third degree, against a person less than fourteen years old, he or she intentionally causes the death of such person.

Murder in the second degree is a class A-I felony.

how the suspect may have transferred any of these substances or used any of these items during the commission of the crime. A more thorough list of forensic techniques is listed in Figure 15.3.

The facts of the case must support the hypothesis and the criteria for the commission of the specific crime in the penal code. For example, in the state of New York, murder in the second degree can be charged in five circumstances (see box above).

The detective must document the location and behavior of all victims (V), suspects (S), and witnesses (W) immediately before, during, and after the crime. All communications by these participants, including written, oral, landline phone, cell phone, computer, pager, and personal data assistant must be found and verified. Any discrepancies within the timeline of events must be resolved.

Frequently Asked Questions

Q: *What is the most difficult part of hypothesis development and case triage team efforts?*

A: The case triage team consists of a group of professionals from multiple agencies that must be able to work together as a team. Excellent people skills and the establishment of trusting/professional relationships between all members of the team are essential for success.

Q: *What is the most effective strategy used during the hypothesis development discussions?*

A: Members of the CTT must have the authority and resources to provide necessary support to the investigative process. The varied backgrounds and expertise of the team in a positive work culture provide the opportunity for different opinions on how the crime may have occurred. Individual biases and stereotypes are diffused in the case triage team environment.

Laura Lake Residence, 159 Walnut Street, Metroland, New York

CRIME SCENE

The case triage team for the Laura Lake homicide is now assembling for the third time in four weeks. The team has been working together nonstop since the first day of the Laura Lake investigation, and includes the following team members:

- First Responder Patrol Officer—Barry Lasker
- Crime Scene Technician—John Goodspeed
- Forensic Scientist Supervisor—Olivia Johns
- Medical Examiner—Dr. Ali Kumar
- Laboratory Quality Assurance Supervisor—Carol Lent
- Forensic Scientist 3, Latents—Larry Poler
- Forensic Scientist 3, DNA—Sara Herbst
- Forensic Scientist 3, Drugs—Sanjay Predeep
- Detective Lieutenant—Daniel Escobar
- Detective, Homicide Squad—Louis Muscato

The team has gone over all of the statements from neighborhood interviews, family members, and phone and computer messages to no avail. The laboratory results all seem to be routine. No drugs or medications have been found in the toxicology analyses of all bodily fluids and tissues. There is also no evidence of a sexual assault exhibited by the injuries and no sperm or seminal fluid was detected in the victim's clothing or swabs collected during the autopsy.

Detective Lieutenant Escobar has been working in the homicide squad for approximately five years. He was previously assigned to the narcotics division for 10 years and needed a change. His wealth of street contacts makes him a very effective detective. He knows the people on the street and

(continued)

(continued)

CRIME SCENE

they know him. More importantly, he has studied the concept of recidivism and is aware of the power of the electronic databases—CODIS, NIBIN, and AFIS. Detective Escobar realizes that one-half of the convicted offenders commit the same crime again in the same neighborhood.

Sam Livingston is a career burglar with many prior convictions. He has had a serious drug addiction for the past 20 years. Sam's criminal history consists of four terms in the New York State correctional system for a variety of burglary and drug-related offenses. As a result of his convictions, he has had to provide a sample of his saliva. His DNA profile has been entered into the Combined DNA Index System (CODIS). Sam is not a violent person but is increasingly desperate to obtain money to purchase drugs for his habit. If a homeowner attacked him during a burglary, he would defend himself. Sam's addiction is severe and he needs to steal property every day so he can sell or trade the stolen goods for drugs.

Sam Livingston, the main suspect, has not been totally excluded but he does appear to have an alibi for the day the homicide occurred. Sam adamantly denies being at the Lake residence the day of the killing. But he was found to have injuries to his hands that appear to be deep scratches. These could have been caused by the victim in the struggle for her life. Sam states that he has a landscaping job at an estate in the same neighborhood and that he injured his hands while trimming brush with power tools. The owner of the estate confirms that Sam has been working hard on the property over the past several weeks. However, the owner was not present at the estate on the day of the homicide. Therefore, he cannot confirm Sam's presence on that day, nor can he confirm the cause of Sam's injuries.

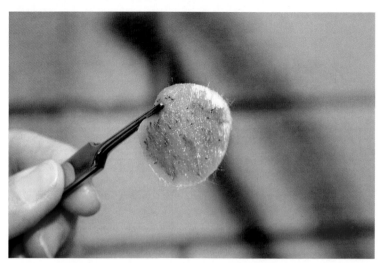

Gunshot residue collection

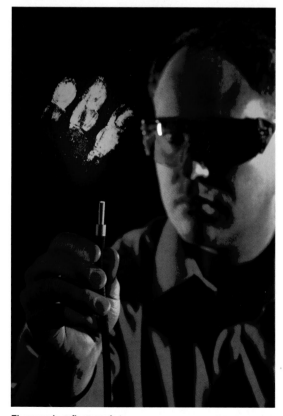

Fluorescing fingerprints

THE CRIME SCENE:
HOW FORENSIC SCIENCE WORKS

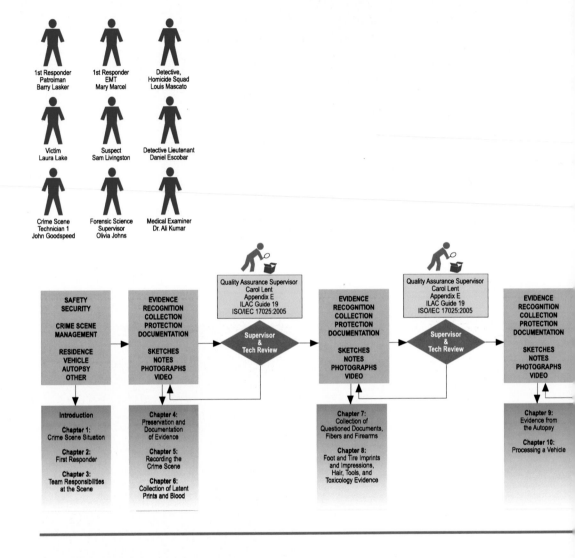

1st Responder Patrolman
Barry Lasker

1st Responder EMT
Mary Marcel

Detective, Homicide Squad
Louis Mascato

Victim
Laura Lake

Suspect
Sam Livingston

Detective Lieutenant
Daniel Escobar

Crime Scene Technician 1
John Goodspeed

Forensic Science Supervisor
Olivia Johns

Medical Examiner
Dr. Ali Kumar

| SAFETY SECURITY | EVIDENCE RECOGNITION COLLECTION PROTECTION DOCUMENTATION | Quality Assurance Supervisor Carol Lent Appendix E ILAC Guide 19 ISO/IEC 17025:2005 | EVIDENCE RECOGNITION COLLECTION PROTECTION DOCUMENTATION | Quality Assurance Supervisor Carol Lent Appendix E ILAC Guide 19 ISO/IEC 17025:2005 | EVIDENCE RECOGNITION COLLECTION PROTECTION DOCUMENTATION |

CRIME SCENE MANAGEMENT

RESIDENCE VEHICLE AUTOPSY OTHER

SKETCHES NOTES PHOTOGRAPHS VIDEO

Supervisor & Tech Review

SKETCHES NOTES PHOTOGRAPHS VIDEO

Supervisor & Tech Review

SKETCHES NOTES PHOTOGRAPHS VIDEO

Introduction

Chapter 1:
Crime Scene Situation

Chapter 2:
First Responder

Chapter 3:
Team Responsibilities at the Scene

Chapter 4:
Preservation and Documentation of Evidence

Chapter 5:
Recording the Crime Scene

Chapter 6:
Collection of Latent Prints and Blood

Chapter 7:
Collection of Questioned Documents, Fibers and Firearms

Chapter 8:
Foot and Tire Imprints and Impressions, Hair, Tools, and Toxicology Evidence

Chapter 9:
Evidence from the Autopsy

Chapter 10:
Processing a Vehicle

EDUCATION & QUALITY & PROFESSIONAL DEVELOPMENT

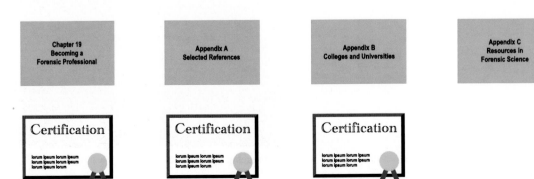

Chapter 19
Becoming a Forensic Professional

Appendix A
Selected References

Appendix B
Colleges and Universities

Appendix C
Resources in Forensic Science

Certification

lorum ipsum lorum ipsum
lorum ipsum lorum ipsum
lorum ipsum lorum

BACHELOR'S DEGREE

Certification

lorum ipsum lorum ipsum
lorum ipsum lorum ipsum
lorum ipsum lorum

GRADUATE DEGREE

Certification

lorum ipsum lorum ipsum
lorum ipsum lorum ipsum
lorum ipsum lorum

PROFESSIONAL DEVELOPMENT

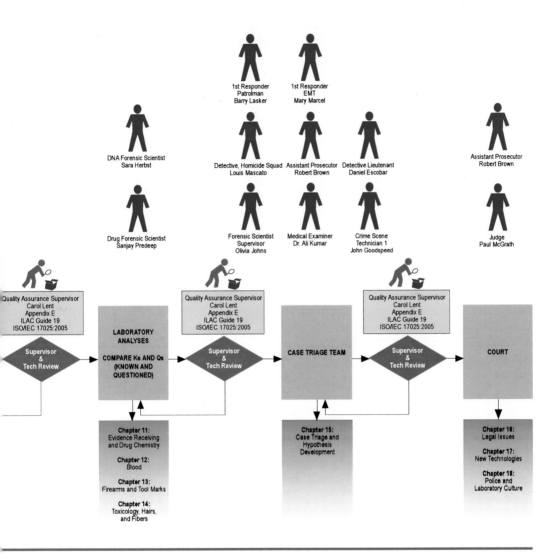

1st Responder
Patrolman
Barry Lasker

1st Responder
EMT
Mary Marcel

DNA Forensic Scientist
Sara Herbst

Detective, Homicide Squad
Louis Mascato

Assistant Prosecutor
Robert Brown

Detective Lieutenant
Daniel Escobar

Assistant Prosecutor
Robert Brown

Drug Forensic Scientist
Sanjay Predeep

Forensic Scientist
Supervisor
Olivia Johns

Medical Examiner
Dr. Ali Kumar

Crime Scene
Technician 1
John Goodspeed

Judge
Paul McGrath

Quality Assurance Supervisor
Carol Lent
Appendix E
ILAC Guide 19
ISO/IEC 17025:2005

Quality Assurance Supervisor
Carol Lent
Appendix E
ILAC Guide 19
ISO/IEC 17025:2005

Quality Assurance Supervisor
Carol Lent
Appendix E
ILAC Guide 19
ISO/IEC 17025:2005

Supervisor
&
Tech Review

LABORATORY
ANALYSES

COMPARE Ks AND Qs
(KNOWN AND
QUESTIONED)

Supervisor
&
Tech Review

CASE TRIAGE TEAM

Supervisor
&
Tech Review

COURT

Chapter 11:
Evidence Receiving
and Drug Chemistry

Chapter 12:
Blood

Chapter 13:
Firearms and Tool Marks

Chapter 14:
Toxicology, Hairs,
and Fibers

Chapter 15:
Case Triage and
Hypothesis
Development

Chapter 16:
Legal Issues

Chapter 17:
New Technologies

Chapter 18:
Police and
Laboratory Culture

Appendix D
Forensic Job Analysis

Appendix E
Quality Assurance
ILAC Guide 19
ISO/IEC 17025:2005

Appendix F
Authors' Forensic
Management Research

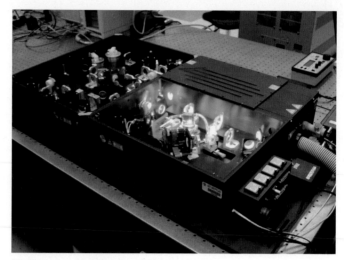

Fiber research with laser

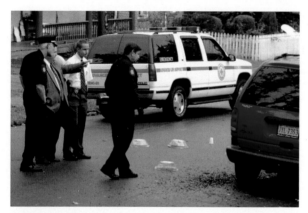

Crime scene team

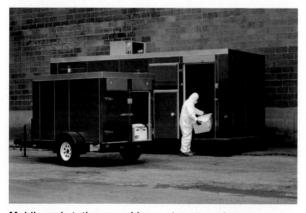

Mobile and stationary evidence storage systems

CHAPTER 16

Legal Issues

fo·ren·sic (fə-rĕn′sĕk, -zĕk)

1. Relating to, used in, or appropriate for courts of law or for public discussion or argumentation.

2. . . . .

3. Relating to the use of science or technology in the investigation and establishment of facts or evidence in a court of law: *a forensic laboratory.* (The American Heritage Dictionary of the English Language, Fourth Edition)

The above definition highlights two major roles of the forensic scientist. First, forensic scientists collect and analyze evidence in support of legal, primarily criminal, investigations. Second, forensic scientists frequently appear as witnesses in court to present the conclusions derived from their analysis of that evidence. This chapter discusses aspects of both roles.

Legal Issues in the Gathering of Forensic Evidence

For the most part, determinations of the legality of searches that lead to forensic evidence lie outside the expertise of the forensic scientist. That said, in many jurisdictions forensic scientists directly engaged in the collection of evidence must have a thorough grounding in the legal requirements for conducting those searches. This section is not intended to represent a complete description of any area of law. Forensic scientists must discuss legal issues with local prosecutors or police officers trained in the collection of evidence.

The Fourth Amendment to the United States Constitution provides the following:

> The right of the people to be secure in their persons, houses, papers, and effects, against unreasonable searches and seizures, shall not be violated, and no Warrants shall issue, but upon probable cause, supported by Oath or affirmation, and particularly describing the place to be searched, and the persons or things to be seized.

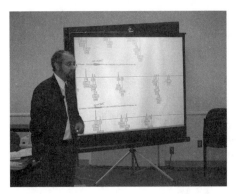

Prosecutor in court

Over the years, the courts have intertwined the amendment's two clauses. As a result, American courts presumptively require the issuance of a search warrant or some other form of court order prior to the seizure of evidence. In general, search of a suspect's home may only occur following the issuance of a search warrant.

Requirements for Search Warrant Exceptions

The courts have recognized a number of exceptions to the requirement for a search warrant. These exceptions often come into play in criminal investigations, resulting in the seizure of evidence subject to forensic analysis.

Search Incident to Arrest

Police may search lawfully arrested subjects and seize any evidence recovered from them or from their immediate area.

Consent

Authorities may search areas for which the owner has voluntarily consented to a search. The scope of the search is limited to the extent of the consent. Note that consent is very frequently the means by which evidence is secured from victims or cooperative witnesses.

Automobiles

Given the mobility of automobiles and the consequent likelihood of the destruction of evidence when a vehicle is allowed to leave a location, the courts have recognized a limited authority for law enforcement to search vehicles. An officer who has probable cause to believe that a vehicle contains evidence may search that vehicle as long as there is some likelihood that the vehicle may be removed during the delay necessary to obtain a search warrant. The time frame for an automobile search is limited. Once a vehicle is in police custody for any appreciable amount of time, law enforcement's ability to conduct a warrantless search evaporates.

Inventory

Containers that come into police possession may be inventoried pursuant to specific police department regulations. The purpose of the inventory is to protect the owner's property against loss, to protect the police against lawsuits resulting from the loss of that property, and to protect the police against dangers, such as concealed bombs. An inventory may not be used as an excuse to conduct a search for evidence.

Exigent Circumstances

If evidence may be destroyed due to an exigency, authorities may seize it without securing a warrant. Fleeing suspects who may destroy evidence in their possession may be pursued and that evidence may be secured, even in areas that would otherwise not be subject to search. The exigent circumstances exception frequently allows for the seizure of a suspect's blood, since biological processes, such as alcohol intoxication, may destroy evidence of crime.

Plain View

Evidence inadvertently observed from a location where an investigator has a lawful presence may be seized. Investigators executing a search warrant for illegal drugs may seize weapons discovered in plain view, even though those weapons are not specified in the search warrant.

Courtroom Presentation

The courtroom represents the greatest difference between the forensic scientist and scientists in other fields. Whether the trier of fact is a jury or a trial judge sitting without a jury, the goal of the forensic scientist is to present the results of forensic analysis in a clear and accurate manner that does not imply bias in favor of either side. To that end, the forensic scientist must keep several things in mind.

Documentation

The rules concerning preservation of documentation and its disclosure among the parties to the case will vary by jurisdiction and by the nature of the case. Whatever those rules might be, the forensic scientist should keep thorough and accurate documentation and should preserve that documentation. Inaccurate or incomplete documentation is often the subject of cross-examination. In addition, lost or destroyed documentation may cause the trier of fact to speculate about what that documentation said.

Preparation

Prior to trial, the forensic scientist should thoroughly review all documentation concerning the scientific analysis that will be the subject of testimony. During that review, mental note should be taken of problems with the documentation, such as missing documentation, inaccuracies in the documentation, or anomalies in the analysis. The forensic scientist should exercise care in taking additional written notes on those issues, since in some jurisdictions the additional written notes may be subject to disclosure.

Before trial, the forensic scientist should meet with the prosecutor. Although many prosecutors strive to educate themselves, the forensic scientist is always in a better position to understand scientific material. As a result, the forensic scientist should prepare to educate the prosecutor about the analysis and results of forensic testing. The forensic scientist should highlight any discrepancies, errors, omissions, or testing anomalies shown in her documentation.

Testimony

The difference between the forensic scientist and other scientists is testimony. Critical issues related to courtroom testimony include qualifications, conduct during testimony, reviewing notes, preparation of visual aids, literature, and calculations.

Qualifications. The forensic scientist should prepare and regularly update her curriculum vitae. In addition, since expert credentials separate the forensic scientist from other witnesses, the forensic scientist should be thoroughly conversant in her own qualifications. Discussion of qualifications should be the forensic scientist's moment to shine, not an occasion for lapses of memory on the witness stand. The young forensic scientist should not be embarrassed by sparse qualifications, but should emphasize her strong points. Areas of expert qualifications include education, employment history, publications, and previous testimony in court or before grand juries.

Conversational Language. The goal of the forensic scientist is to convince the jury of the accuracy of scientific analysis. A jury is much more likely to believe testimony if it is presented in a conversational style. Scientific terms should be discarded in favor of equivalent, nonscientific explanations. For example, rather than the word "analysis," the forensic scientist could choose "testing." Instead of the word "reagents," the scientist can say "chemicals." Rather than the word "migrate" to describe electrophoresis, the scientist could use "travel" or "move."

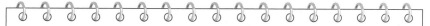

During a mock trial exercise, a student forensic scientist described a process in which chemicals "get happy." While certainly conversational, this language does not accurately convey the nature of the analysis. Such inaccuracies should be avoided.

Reducing scientific terminology to conversational language can be difficult. The forensic scientist should consider how to describe the work to a friend or relative who is not involved in science. Conversational language does not mean inaccurate language. The forensic scientist should choose language that correctly conveys the nature and results of scientific testing. Conversational analogies designed to illustrate the nature of scientific testing in layman's terms should be developed and rehearsed.

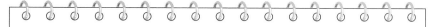

Simple analogies can be used to describe complex phenomena. For example, a conversational analogy could include "boxcars" to describe simple repeat sequences of STR loci. "A tennis ball and a beach ball" can illustrate the relative strengths of the walls of a sperm cell and an epithelial cell in a differential extraction.

Eye Contact. Since the forensic scientist's goal is to convince the jury, she should look at the jury. Eye contact conveys sincerity. The experienced prosecutor will often help by positioning himself in the courtroom so that the forensic scientist witness is forced to look toward the jury. There is a happy medium between looking at the jury in response to every question and looking robotic. Turning the head toward the jury to give a one-word answer can look stilted, and should be reserved for longer explanations.

Direct and Cross-Examination. The party calling a witness conducts direct examination. Then the opposing party conducts cross-examination. The calling party may then ask questions on redirect examination, followed by recross-examination, and the process may continue in that fashion until both parties have completed examining the witness. There is a fundamental difference between the nature of direct examination—that is, examination conducted by the party calling a witness—and cross-examination, conducted by the opposing party. Television courtroom dramas often show attorneys objecting that "counsel is leading the witness," without describing the concept of a "leading" question. A leading question is one that suggests the answer, and may generally not be used by the party calling a witness. On the other hand, the party cross-examining a witness is permitted to use leading questions, and good cross-examiners will use them almost completely. Thus, for example, the question "What color was the traffic light?" is nonleading, since it suggests no answer and the witness is free to provide the requested information. On the other hand, the question "The traffic light was red, right?" is leading since it clearly suggests the answer the examiner seeks. Leading questions must still be answered accurately, and the forensic scientist should not be taken in by the phrasing of the question. Note that nonleading does not necessarily mean broadly phrased. Questioners can ask nonleading questions that focus on specific facts. Some prosecutors will ask forensic scientists narrow questions, moving them through a direct examination in baby steps. Some prosecutors will ask very broad questions, and expect

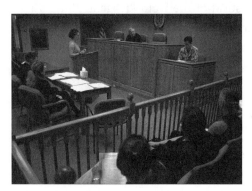

Typical courtroom

the forensic scientist to provide all the details. The forensic scientist should be prepared for both types of direct examination.

Refreshing Recollection. No witness is required to completely remember every detail of the facts they are to testify about. Given the complexity of forensic science, it is likely that the forensic scientist witness will forget some detail of her analysis. If that happens, the forensic scientist may simply ask the court for permission to review her notes so that she can provide accurate testimony. Courts will frequently dispense with the requirement of asking for permission, but the forensic scientist should at first defer to the court for guidance. Of course, forensic scientists should thoroughly review the case before testifying to minimize the number of times needed to refresh memory.

Visual Aids. The forensic scientist may be called upon to prepare visual aids for the prosecutor. These visual aids include charts that illustrate the results of forensic testing. Presentation software, such as Microsoft Power-Point, is often used to present material in court. Many forensic laboratories will have the facilities to prepare such courtroom presentations. The forensic scientist should be conversant in the various technologies in order to assist in the preparation of those visual aids.

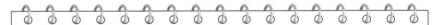

Daubert Decision: 1993 United States Supreme Court, *Daubert* v. *Dow Pharmaceuticals, Inc.*

Daubert established new standards regarding scientific legitimacy and the limitations of professional scope with respect to the court system. The following are considered:

- Has the scientific theory or technique been subjected to peer review and publication?
- What is the known or potential error rate?
- What are the expert's qualifications and stature in the scientific community?
- Can the technique and its results be explained with sufficient clarity and simplicity so that the court and the jury can understand its plain meaning?

Cross-Examination with Literature. Defense attorneys frequently use published writings as sources for cross-examination questions. Before an attorney can quote from a published writing, the expert witness must admit that the writing is "authoritative." Once that admission is made, the expert witness may be cross-examined with any material in the writing. The forensic scientist should avoid admitting that a specific source is "authoritative." At a minimum, the forensic scientist should be thoroughly conversant in the writing before making that admission.

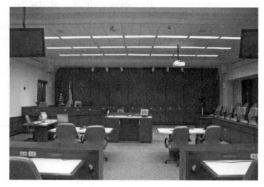

Courtroom

Calculations. Forensic work often requires detailed numerical calculations. Attorneys often ask the forensic scientist to perform calculations on the witness stand. This should be avoided, since an inaccuracy can undermine the witness's credibility. If asked to perform calculations, the witness should defer, asking the court for a recess to perform calculations outside the jury's presence, using other resource material if available.

Frequently Asked Questions

Q: *Is there a minimum amount of experience the forensic scientist must have before he may testify in court?*

A: No. The forensic scientist may be called to testify about the first case that he handled. He must be prepared to testify from the beginning of his career.

Q: *Will the forensic scientist ever be called upon to prepare a search warrant?*

A: Probably not. In general, prosecutors and police are trained to prepare search warrants, and the forensic scientist will not be required to do so. The forensic scientist may, however, be called upon to sign a sworn statement in support of a search warrant.

Q: *Is there a minimum qualification level before a forensic scientist may testify?*

A: Legally, no. As long as the forensic scientist is qualified to discuss the area, he may testify about it. There may be standards within the particular scientific field that must be met before the forensic scientist performs the work, but failure to meet those standards would not alone preclude the forensic scientist from testifying.

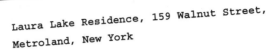

Laura Lake Residence, 159 Walnut Street, Metroland, New York

CRIME SCENE

Defense attorney Howard Chapin, prosecutor Robert Brown, and judge Paul McGrath have known each other for years. Howard worked with Robert in the prosecutor's office for 10 years before he decided to go into private practice. Paul had worked as the district attorney for Metroland for 22 years, and was recently elected county court judge. All of the attorneys avoided science while obtaining their education at the local state university and law school. However, they have all managed to keep up with the rapid changes in forensic science using professional development programs provided by the state. The state judicial training institute has done a remarkable job in providing continuing learning credits with yearly DNA seminars. Robert makes sure that all documents related to the investigation and laboratories are provided to the defense in a timely manner.

Judge McGrath has been sitting as the county court judge for five years. He has presided over several homicide cases that were relatively simple and did not entail any evidence. He knows this case will have several types of DNA and he is going to enroll in a continuing education credit class on forensic science. There has been a recent Supreme Court decision (*Daubert* v. *Dow Pharmaceuticals, Inc.*) that has revolutionized the courtroom, and placed the burden on the judges for monitoring acceptance of scientific testimony. The judge is now the "gatekeeper" of scientific evidence in the courtroom.

The lack of any victim's DNA from blood on the suspect's shoes was very problematic in the early stages of the investigation.

CHAPTER 17

New Forensic Technology

Laboratory information management systems (LIMS) are the essential foundation of the forensic laboratory. New technology in the forensic sciences helps to develop information systems involving a wide spectrum of databases and software applications. This provides a reliable and increasingly effective network for transferring information between the forensic team, detectives, precincts, departments, states, and countries. For example, handheld BlackBerry devices aid communication between the lab and detectives at the crime

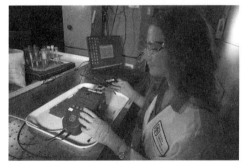

New technology

scene. This chapter reviews new forensic techniques and provides examples of the influence of technology in the criminal justice community.

Prior to the availability of computer-based databases, detectives submitted bullets or bullet casings to the laboratory, and ballistic examiners matched the bullet directly to the evidence from a specific known weapon. It was only through serendipity that a bullet could be matched to a separate criminal case or weapon, without a specific request by the detective. Similarly, latent print comparisons across cases or jurisdictions occurred only occasionally. In these rare instances, a forensic scientist or detective

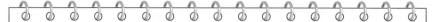

The Importance of Linking Cases

New computerized laboratory information management systems (LIMS) routinely look for linkages between cases. The case below is an example of the dedication of experienced scientists and investigators linking many cases over many years *without LIMS.*

Marybeth Tinning, convicted of killing her infant daughter and long suspected in the death of her other children, was denied parole in March 2007. The parole board criticized Tinning, 64, for refusing to acknowledge her responsibility for her daughter's death and for showing no remorse. During interviews, Tinning stated that she did not believe that she would harm her child but could not recall exactly what occurred.

In letters to the parole board, district attorneys who prosecuted the case stated that Tinning also admitted to trying to kill her husband, Joseph, and killing her son, Nathan, and six of her other children between the mid-1970s and 1985. Authorities have stated that Tinning probably killed eight of her nine children. Unlike other cases where a parent kills children in one incident, these events took place over a period of nearly 14 years.

would remember a specific peculiarity common to two or more cases and then compare the case files to confirm the association.

Historically, hard copies of case files were stored in file cabinets and archived in large warehouse systems. Index cards were maintained by detectives for ready reference and name checks in the home patrol area. A bound journal was used to write down sequential case numbers for all criminal complaints and requests for assistance received by the department. The forensic laboratory maintained a similar logbook to record all evidence submitted and returned.

These logbooks and index cards are now replaced with sophisticated laboratory information management systems (LIMS). New information technology is classified into a global law enforcement network containing a subset of forensic databases. Detectives and scientists investigating both current and cold cases use these systems. Many databases are available for information searches (see appendix C for Web links to these databases). The FBI supports a Criminal Justice Information System (CJIS), which provides the backbone for sharing information between all law enforcement agencies. CJIS includes several systems.

Integrated Automated Fingerprint Identification System (IAFIS)

IAFIS collects all 10-print cards developed from arrestees and the latent prints developed from crime scenes. These prints are routinely correlated to provide matches or exclusions. IAFIS, the largest biometric database in the world, contains over 47 million electronic 10-print cards. All U.S. states have their own statewide automated fingerprint identification system (AFIS), and they contribute prints to IAFIS. Digital images are taken from the latent fingerprints and standardized biometric identifiers are electronically embedded on the latent print to allow comparison to other fingerprints.

Law Enforcement Online (LEO)

LEO is a secure network designed specifically for use by law enforcement to communicate with other agencies. LEO contains sensitive but not classified information for use in criminal investigations. Law enforcement professionals must apply for access in order to use LEO.

National Instant Criminal Background Check System (NICS)

NICS was established in 1993 with the passage of the Brady Handgun Violence Prevention Act. NICS requires federal firearm licensees to initiate a background check on all individuals who make a request to purchase a weapon.

National Crime Information Center (NCIC)

The central database for tracking crime-related information in the United States is NCIC. NCIC is maintained by the FBI and linked with similar systems in each state. Data is received from federal, state, and local law enforcement agencies, including non–law enforcement agencies, such as motor vehicle registration and licensing authorities, and includes the following:

- *Enhanced Name Search* provides searches of convicted offenders using phonetically similar names or derivatives of names.
- *Fingerprints* searches the right index finger on all wanted and missing persons.
- *Probation and Parole* contains searchable records of convicted offenders currently being supervised by probation and parole departments.

- *Mugshots* provides one mugshot, fingerprint, and other identifying information for searches and comparisons.

Uniform Crime Reporting/National Incident Based Reporting System (UCR/NIBRS)

UCR/NIBRS is an incident-based reporting system that collects, compiles, analyzes, and publishes all crime data for the United States. Specific facts about serious crimes are gathered and reported in the NIBRS system.

National Integrated Ballistic Information Network (NIBIN)

The federal Bureau of Alcohol, Tobacco, Firearms and Explosives (ATF) supports the NIBIN database. ATF works with local, state, and federal agencies to install and maintain a network of all law enforcement agencies that have forensic ballistic laboratories. As discussed in detail in chapter 7 and chapter 13, ballistic laboratories process firearm evidence in criminal cases for the operability, identification, and microscopic comparison of projectiles and cartridge casings. Digital photographs from cartridges and casings are stored in a database for comparison. The unique markings from the firing pin, breech marks, and ejectors are imprinted upon the cartridge case. The microscopic tool marks from the lands and grooves in the barrel are imprinted upon the projectiles. These unique markings are used to compare questioned

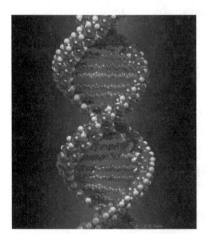

DNA helix

and known projectiles and bullets to known weapons. The NIBIN database represents more than 200 sites throughout the United States, Guam, Puerto Rico, and the Virgin Islands. Over 3,400 leads have been generated from 180,000 bullets and casings in NIBIN's database.

Combined DNA Index System (CODIS)

CODIS allows federal, state, and local crime labs to electronically exchange and compare DNA profiles in order to link crimes to each other and to convicted offenders. The database is managed by the FBI. The primary performance measure in CODIS is a hit or "investigation aided." When a hit occurs, the CODIS custodian confirms

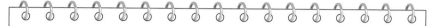

Cold Case Solved with CODIS

The case below is a good example of how new technology and the CODIS database system solve old homicide cases.

On July 4, 1992, the body of 15-year-old Sean Googin was found floating in Cazenovia Lake in upstate New York. Even though the body had been submerged in water, the autopsy recovered evidence of a sexual attack. Over 2,500 leads were followed, including an effort to locate all known pedophiles in local counties, but all suspects were eliminated.

The forensic science team at the New York State Police Forensics Unit developed a full DNA profile from the cold case of Sean Googin. In 1999 Jeffrey Clark was arrested for a separate sexual offense and his DNA was put into CODIS. Clark's DNA was matched to DNA obtained from the Googin crime scene. The investigation was reopened, Clark was arrested, and he pleaded guilty to second-degree murder in his full confession. He was sentenced to 23 years to life in prison.

the identity and qualifying offense of the convicted offender. Additional confirmatory analysis of the DNA sample is performed for quality control. The two laboratories are notified that the system has identified the link. The labs then contact their respective police departments and prosecutors to inform them of the hit. The hit serves as *reasonable cause* to collect a final confirmatory DNA sample from the convicted offender. The confirmatory DNA sample is compared to the actual evidence in the case as a quality control check for the entire CODIS system.

CODIS compares known convicted offenders (Ks) and unknown forensic samples from crime scenes (Qs) from all 50 states. Figure 17.1 shows the relationship between the national (federal), state, and local DNA systems. Table 17.1 shows that through February 2007, 46,325 investigations have been aided using CODIS.

Criminal history information indicates CODIS-qualifying offenses and that a DNA profile is available in the CODIS system. Criminal history records indicate if the inmate or released offender has been convicted of a CODIS offense and needs to provide a CODIS sample. Other databases also track recidivistic sexual offenders; their known locations are controlled by probation and parole officers.

FIGURE 17.1 *CODIS Structure*

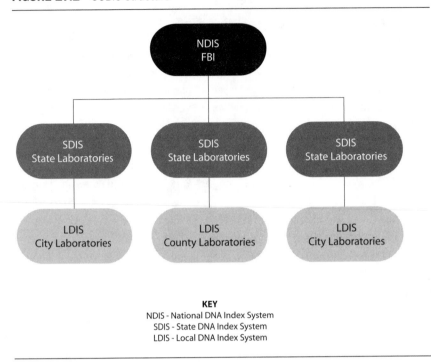

KEY
NDIS - National DNA Index System
SDIS - State DNA Index System
LDIS - Local DNA Index System

FIGURE 17.2 *CODIS Map*

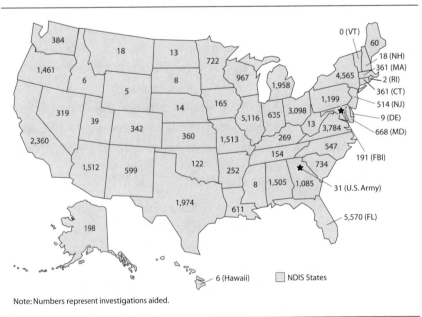

Note: Numbers represent investigations aided.

TABLE 17.1 *CODIS Hits, Through February 2007*

State	Investigations Aided*	State	Investigations Aided
Alabama	1,505	Missouri	1,513
Alaska	198	Montana	18
Arizona	1,512	Nebraska	14
Arkansas	252	Nevada	319
California	2,360	New Hampshire	18
Colorado	342	New Jersey	514
Connecticut	361	New Mexico	599
Delaware	9	New York	4,565
District of Columbia	191	North Carolina	547
	(FBI Lab)	North Dakota	13
Florida	5,570	Ohio	3,098
Georgia	1,085	Oklahoma	122
	(31 U.S. Army Crime Lab)	Oregon	1,461
Hawaii	6	Pennsylvania	1,199
Idaho	6	Rhode Island	2
Illinois	5,116	South Carolina	734
Indiana	635	South Dakota	8
Iowa	165	Tennessee	154
Kansas	360	Texas	1,974
Kentucky	269	Utah	39
Louisiana	511	Vermont	0
Maine	60	Virginia	3,784
Maryland	668	Washington	384
Massachusetts	361	West Virginia	13
Michigan	1,958	Wisconsin	967
Minnesota	772	Wyoming	5
Mississippi	8		

Source: www.fbi.gov

* "Investigations Aided" is a metric that tracks the number of criminal investigations where CODIS has added value to the investigative process.

Linkages between sexual offender registries and convicted offender DNA databases are becoming more sophisticated in that they focus technology on the most probative area of violent crime. For example, police chiefs need to know the status and location of all repeat sexual offenders in their geopolitical jurisdiction and whether there is a DNA profile available from a DNA data bank. In addition, the police need to follow up on local sexual offenders with unknown addresses or convicted offenders who have not provided a DNA sample. These databases are useful to the extent that they aid in monitoring convicted offenders and their movements.

DNA Database Performance Metrics

In business, financial analysts compare publicly traded companies in the same industry using key ratios of performance. The key performance measure for the CODIS system is the "hit" or "investigation aided." Determining the actual outcome of the DNA hit report is inherently complex in that the hit could provide linkage to another case (case-to-case linkage without an offender) or match a specific convicted offender.

The CODIS system has matured to the point that established performance metrics can be developed using 2005 data from *www.fbi.gov* and *www.us.census.gov.* Performance measures allow comparison between similar laboratories. These performance measures are not all-inclusive. Key variables such as number of total personnel, amount of local and federal funding, and capacity of facilities and equipment would add value to a benchmark analysis of the CODIS program. Private industry uses these types of ratios to compare management efficiency, such as product or service unit per employee or return on investment. Similarly, forensic science must continue to establish reliable and valid performance measures for its multiple stakeholders. Tables 17.2 through 17.9 are examples of CODIS benchmarks between states. Policy makers should monitor these performance ratios to detect positive trends and reward top performers.

CODIS Funding

The CODIS program is funded in a variety of ways by local, state, and federal levels of government. The FBI provides oversight, research support, and the infrastructure to maintain the CODIS network and develop casework analytical methods.

Formula grants use statewide population statistics or a national percentage of violent crimes in a state as a guide for funding distribution. A major performance metric of the CODIS program is the number of investigations aided by the total CODIS program. The National Institute of Justice (NIJ) DNA Capacity Program Enhancement Grant (June 2005) is a formula (number of violent offenses reported to FBI) grant that will distribute

TABLE 17.2 *Top 10 States Forensic Samples per Capita*

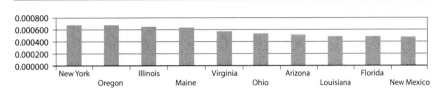

TABLE 17.3 *Top 10 States Forensic Samples*

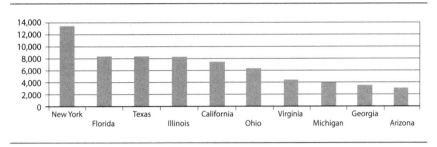

TABLE 17.4 *Top 10 States Investigations Aided per Forensic Sample*

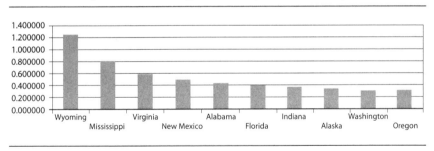

TABLE 17.5 *Top 10 States Investigations Aided*

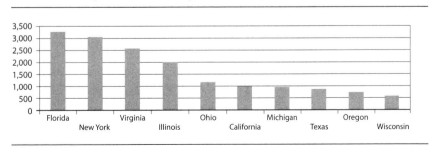

TABLE 17.6   *Top 10 States Number of CODIS Labs*

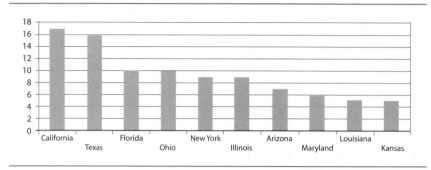

TABLE 17.7   *Top 10 States Offending Profiles*

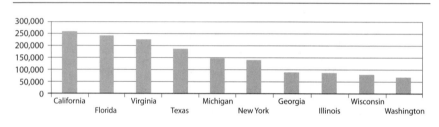

TABLE 17.8   *Top 10 States Offender Profiles per Capita*

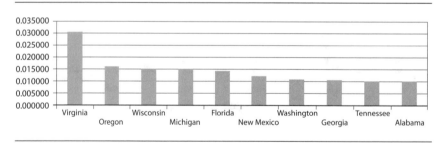

TABLE 17.9   *Top 10 States Investigations Aided by Convicted Offender Samples*

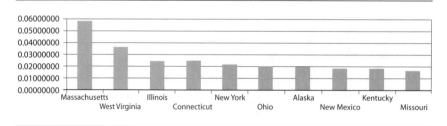

TABLE 17.10 *Top 10 States Funding NIJ Capacity Formula Grants*

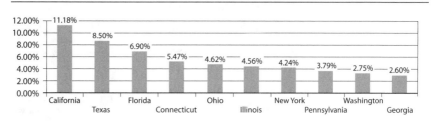

$31.5 million to improve laboratory DNA capacity. Table 17.10 shows how funding is distributed through the formula percentage. Table 17.4 shows the top 10 states by CODIS hits.

The following are the states listed with the highest frequency in the top 10 states of all key ratios of performance:

- Florida
- New York
- Illinois
- Virginia

Analyses of the CODIS programs in Florida, New York, Illinois, and Virginia reveal that they are exemplars and model programs. Development of a model program would include both tangible (facilities, equipment) and intangible (personnel, education) assets. Larger databases take advantage of economy of scale and increased efficiency. Their performance metrics for success in the CODIS system are recognized as models in the forensic community. Smaller states can collaborate with each other to leverage these advantages.

Computer Crime and Digital Evidence

Computer crime analysis and digital evidence is the new forensic discipline. The American Society of Crime Laboratory Directors/Laboratory Accreditation Board (ASCLD/LAB) has approved computer crime as an accredited discipline as part of the ASCLD/LAB accreditation process. Accreditation of computer crime is now voluntary and is not yet an essential part of the accreditation process. This is normally done to provide a transition period for a new scientific discipline. Laboratories face a challenge when designing competency and proficiency tests for the tasks performed in computer crime analyses. Training, professional development, and academic curriculums in computer crime are now gaining support in academic institutions. Partnerships are being formed between forensic laboratories, colleges, and private industry.

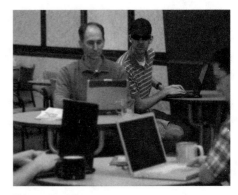

Computer crime

Computer crime and digital evidence can be divided among four major categories:

- Copying and extracting data
- Support for computer crime investigations
- Intrusions and information assurance
- Audio/video enhancements and analyses

Copying and Extraction

Copying and extraction involves analysis of the full set of digital media storage devices. All information pertinent to a criminal investigation is collected, printed, and archived for use in criminal investigation. The specific techniques used do not compromise the data, chain of custody, or integrity of the data for use in criminal court proceedings. Digital storage devices consist of hard drives, floppy diskettes, compact discs, personal digital assistants, cell phones, global positioning systems, tape systems, and MP3 storage devices. Routine repairs are also performed on storage systems that have failed or have been damaged.

Major Crimes Digital Evidence

Major crimes digital evidence units specialize in the recognition, collection, and protection of digital evidence for the prosecution of specific computer crimes. For example, cases that involve downloading and distributing child pornography or cases with sexual predators are now routinely investigated by law enforcement. Computer crimes typically can involve one or more of the following: theft, fraud, violent crime, sexual assault, misuse of government computers, password identification, and peer-to-peer network tracking.

Intrusions and Information Assurance Solutions

Intrusions and information assurance solutions analyzes and monitors computer networks to detect any unauthorized intrusions, theft of data, or virus contamination. Procedures to visualize and mine data are also used to analyze large amounts of data efficiently. Firewall performance is maintained and unauthorized embedded coding is detected and removed to protect sensitive law enforcement network systems. Blind proficiency tests are designed to confirm the effectiveness and performance of existing firewall and security protection systems.

Audio and Video Forensics Solutions

Audio and video forensics solutions performs forensics analysis of virtually all types of audio and visual digital files. Files are enhanced to reduce noise and increase video clarity. Common types of evidence include surveillance, security recordings, and digital photographs.

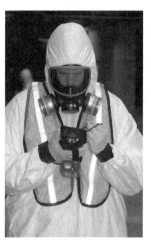

First responder with PDA and Haz-mat gear

CJIS, AFIS, CODIS, NIBIN, and the new forensic discipline of computer crime analysis have dramatically changed the techniques and operation of the forensic laboratory. Forensic analytical instruments are totally operated by computer. Electronic databases routinely compare thousands of fingerprints, DNA profiles, and ballistic images. Laboratory information management systems have replaced evidence logbooks with bar codes and paperless office document management systems. Computerized systems have increased the efficiency and speed of the forensic laboratory analyses. Forensic scientists of the future will implement robotics, miniaturization, and new DNA techniques, such as RNA and mitochondrial DNA analyses. The challenge for the forensic laboratory of the future will be to keep up with technology through the support and nurturing of a learning culture in the laboratory. Education, professional development, and professional contacts within the forensic community are essential for the forensic scientist to keep abreast of the latest technology.

Frequently Asked Questions

Q: *What type of training or education is available to prepare for a career in digital evidence or computer crime?*

A: Forensic computer scientists possess excellent computer or information technology skills. Many have advanced degrees in computer science or database management. A good place to start is to obtain a business degree with a specialty in information science. This preparation is directly applicable to the tasks performed by forensic computer scientists.

Q: *What is multidiscipline analysis?*

A: Computer crimes often involve multiple disciplines within the forensic sciences. For example, case evidence might be evaluated for the presence of both fingerprints and DNA of the perpetrator. The surface of the keyboard and debris found under the keys are excellent sources of human DNA source material.

CHAPTER 18

Police and Laboratory Culture

rganizational culture is the shared beliefs and values communicated by leaders to employees. Organizational culture can be intangible and difficult to describe. But culture is important in that dysfunctional values and beliefs may drive good employees out of the organization. In addition, it is important to assess employee "fit" with organizational culture at entry. Ongoing monitoring of culture is needed to make sure that it is in alignment with the goals of the organization.

Employee knowledge, skills, and abilities are usually assessed during phases of the selection system and developed during in-house training programs. Police recruits have varied educational backgrounds: some recruits possess academic degrees that include high school, associate's, bachelor's, master's, and doctoral-level degrees. All recruits undergo rigorous training in a

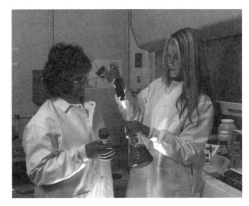

Training

formal academy that consists of at least six months in most jurisdictions. Specialty schools also exist for assignments such as narcotics and other unique law enforcement units. Very few police officers possess a degree

FIGURE 18.1 *Typical Forensic Laboratory Organization Chart*

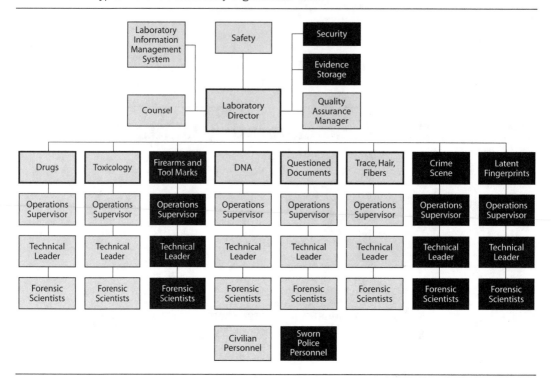

in science or have a background in technology. It is a rare case when an individual with a science degree, through serendipity, finds a career in law enforcement.

The duties performed by employees also contribute to organizational culture. Duties must be in alignment with the existing skill sets and educational background of employees. A thorough job analysis helps to create the list of duties required for the jobs performed daily in the police department. Many support tasks require advanced degrees in technology, finance, communications, aircraft operations, and maintenance. A lack of sworn officers with advanced scientific background and education has increased the importance of hiring civilians with specialized skills so that police departments can provide the best law enforcement and laboratory services.

The American Society of Crime Laboratory Directors/Laboratory Accreditation Board (ASCLD/LAB) lists 330 labs that are accredited. Distribution consists of 180 state, 100 local, 22 federal, 10 international, and 18 private laboratories. All are part of a law enforcement agency, except for 18 private labs. The directory of the ASCLD lists 558 members; 400 of these

FIGURE 18.2 *Typical Police Organization Chart*

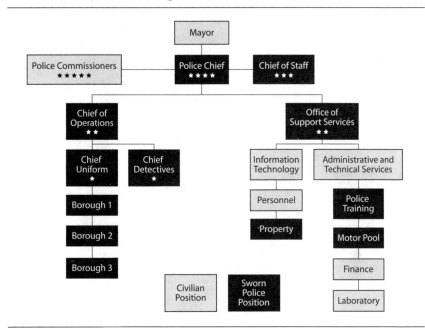

directors reside in labs controlled by police departments. Remaining ASCLD members are from academia, are retired, or supervise private labs.

Most public forensic laboratories are embedded within law enforcement organizations, such as police departments. Figure 18.1 provides a typical forensic laboratory structure and Figure 18.2 provides a typical police department structure. Police departments are paramilitary-type organizations that function within a strict hierarchical structure. Decisions come from the top and may take weeks or months. All communication including orders and assignments move top down from higher authority to line staff. Two factors that determine an individual's authority and respect in a police organization are time served (tenure) and grade level. Number of years on the job and rank are used to determine who will lead a particular unit.

Corporate failure in the private sector is often attributed to cultural factors. For example, an organization may be described as having a "culture of conformity" or a "culture of failure." In addition, "clash" of cultures is often used to describe why mergers between two companies fail. Police and laboratories may have their own clash of cultures. Table 18.1 lists several aspects of contrasting culture in the respective organizations.

TABLE 18.1 *Comparison of Police and Laboratory Organizational Culture*

Organization Culture Variable	Police Department and Sworn Personnel	Laboratory and Civilian Personnel
Core Competency	Police specialize in law enforcement, investigating criminal offenses; at times a dangerous job. Testimony is required.	Forensic laboratory specializes in scientific analyses, analytical chemistry, instrumental analyses, and testimony.
Corrective Action vs. Opportunity for Improvement	Unacceptable actions often lead to disciplinary outcomes.	Unacceptable actions lead to opportunity for improvements. May lead to disciplinary action when they involve integrity.
Decision Making	Very little opportunity for decision making. Actions predetermined by specific policies and procedural manuals and training. When decisions needed, a very hierarchical bureaucratic structure slowly responds to the incident.	Decisions are made by predetermined specific policies and procedural manuals and training. When decisions needed, the scientist can deviate from policy with sound scientific judgment.
Demographics	Applicants for police department must pass entrance examination or civil service test. Minimum education is required.	Applicants for scientific positions must pass civil service examination (in public laboratories). Scientific personnel possess advanced science degrees and may have research backgrounds.
Distribution of Information	Information delivered vertically (top down) in the hierarchical structure of the organization. Very little information is delivered officially via horizontal methods.	Information is delivered directly from source to the individual in need. The environment is less filtered, with the information being delivered to the scientist on the bench in a timely manner.
Improvement Incentives	Reactive culture. In general, no incentives provided.	Proactive culture. In general, opportunities for improvement ideas are encouraged by ISO/IEC 17025:2005 Quality Management Systems.
Learning Environment	Professional development opportunities, education, and in-house training are secondary to the primary law enforcement responsibilities.	Professional development, education, and in-house training are essential to stay abreast of new scientific developments.
Performance Expectations	Police operate all assignments with hard or categorical timelines and dates. Completion dates are set for all tasks, with consequences if dates not met.	Laboratory finds hard completion dates difficult to complete as laboratory analyses are dependent upon many variables not in the scientist's control. Laboratory analyses are also subjected to unexplained anomalies that cause unexpected results.

TABLE 18.1 *Comparison of Police and Laboratory Organizational Culture (continued)*

Organization Culture Variable	Police Department and Sworn Personnel	Laboratory and Civilian Personnel
Performance Incentives	Performance is rewarded through ceremonies or written awards.	Performance is rewarded with patents rights and monetary rewards if revenues increase.
Response to Change	Police organization requires extensive study before adopting any changes in protocols or procedures.	Laboratory is flexible and adaptable to change. Scientific techniques and instrumentation change rapidly.
Response to Crisis	Crisis is responded to with categorical action steps designed to stop the crisis situation quickly in a controlled environment.	The laboratory will respond to a crisis in a measured manner consistent with scientific policies.
Salary Structure	Salary structure designed by multiple labor/management contracts. Recent arbitration decisions have significantly increased police pay.	Scientific unions are small in comparison to police unions and have not been successful raising salaries of scientists.
Stability	Police personnel stay on the job for at least 20 years to earn a pension. Very few individuals leave once vested in retirement system.	Laboratory personnel need to stay with job for pension, but may have to stay for 25 to 30 years before they are vested.
Tolerance for Errors	Police departments have *low* tolerance for errors and progressively serious consequences, including dismissal or criminal charges.	Laboratories have *no* tolerance for errors and progressively serious consequences, including dismissal or criminal charges.
Values and Beliefs	Values and beliefs are generally conservative, consistent with most law enforcement organizations.	Laboratory personnel value the scientific method and unbiased data. The scientist may be liberal or conservative.

Police organizations also use competitive promotional exams to select key job titles. For example, competitive exams are often used to select initial applicants, as well as sergeant, lieutenant, and captain positions. A subjective appointment process is used to select individuals within competitive ranks. Sworn personnel (police take an oath and swear to uphold the laws of the geopolitical service region) work side by side with unsworn personnel (civilians). Sworn and civilian personnel are represented by different labor organizations. Information, policies, and procedures are defined in strict detail in task-oriented manuals.

In general, police organizational culture encourages conservative values and beliefs and an aversion to risk-taking behaviors. Notably, only significant events lead to change in policy and procedure. In contrast, scientists are encouraged to develop new ideas and thinking as part of their education and training. Scientists possess advanced education, technical expertise, and specialty skills such as aircraft, automotive maintenance, information technology, and laboratory forensics. These specialty positions are often occupied by civilian personnel who possess advanced science degrees.

The mixture of law enforcement personnel with civilian scientific personnel forms a unique organizational climate that often leads to a stressful environment. Differences in education, salary, job competencies, and values accentuate the inherent pressures related to productivity and quality of the forensic scientific analyses. The forensic scientist must not commit any errors. However, all scientists are human and will commit errors, either small or large. The work of a forensic scientist directly affects the lives of victims and suspects. Errors will lead to consequences, some as severe as dismissal or at the very least, discipline. The scientist must be detail oriented and possess excellent organizational skills. Supervisors and technical leaders review all work multiple times before a report is issued to the criminal justice system.

Laura Lake Residence, 159 Walnut Street, Metroland, New York

Laboratory forensic scientists have processed all items of evidence looking for any fingerprints or blood from Sam Livingston at the crime scene. None were found. Sam's clothing and vehicle were processed for any blood from Laura Lake, with negative results. The laboratory dedicated several scientists to work this case and they have analyzed over 100 items of evidence attempting to identify either Sam's fingerprints or blood found at the crime scene, or known samples from the victim, Laura Lake, in Sam's vehicle.

EMT Mary Marcel is particularly distraught, knowing that she may have compromised the significant blood spatter evidence at the scene. When she arrived at the scene, Mary was concerned that victim Laura Lake was still alive. Mary rushed to apply CPR, and use a portable defibrillator. Since the victim was still warm, Mary thought that there may be a chance to save the victim. Her job is to save lives. Even though she has been trained in the preservation of evidence, Mary unknowingly stepped in and destroyed several bloody footprints next to the body of the victim. These may have been made by the perpetrator.

The shoes confiscated from the suspect have several bloody smears and blood drops. One particular blood drop came from the top of the shoe. It is consistent with a low velocity, vertical droplet. This could have been from the suspect's hand wounds, allegedly caused by working as a landscaper. The DNA lab works quickly to process the blood drops from the top of the shoe. They are from suspect Sam Livingston. Sam's alibi is holding up.

Carol Lent, quality assurance supervisor, has been a serologist with the laboratory for 25 years. Recently Carol was promoted

(continued)

(continued)

CRIME SCENE

to a newly created supervisor position. She has seen the biology section progress from the old ABO blood typing to the new technology of DNA. Polymerase chain reaction (PCR) obtains DNA profiles from trace or invisible amounts of blood, semen, or saliva. As a serologist, Carol has worked many homicides over the course of her career. The lab had needed one person to take charge of quality assurance in order to prepare the laboratory for the new ISO/IEC 17025:2005 accreditation program. Carol decided that it was time to move into an administrative position in order to contribute to the overall quality of laboratory operations. Carol has the right background for her new supervisory duties as she has attended many accreditation courses and has successfully prepared the lab for several International Standards Organization (ISO) accreditation inspections in the past. It appears that the new forensic scientists in the lab are skilled in DNA analysis since they possess advanced degrees in molecular biology.

But Carol misses casework so she tries to attend case triage team meetings when her schedule permits. Sitting next to EMT Mary Marcel, Carol thinks about the footprints found next to the victim and wishes they had not been obliterated. The photos of the floor at the scene clearly show the presence of another set of shoes, but the imprints in blood could only be matched to Mary Marcel's shoes. The other set of shoe prints do not have enough detail remaining to match to the shoes of suspect Sam Livingston.

Carol asks Detective Lieutenant Daniel Escobar for the photo file. The team has taken over 500 photos of the scene and all items of evidence. Carol wants to see the shoes. Mary's shoes are covered with blood and the imprints are clearly caused by her tread design. Carol next focuses on Sam Livingston's shoes. The round blood drop on the top of the

(continued)

CRIME SCENE

right shoe is very noticeable on the lightly colored shoelaces and shoe top. However, the sides of Sam's shoes and soles are black. Carol asks to have Sam's shoes sent to the clean room in the DNA lab so that she can inspect them more closely.

The next week Carol comes back to the case triage team meeting and announces, "Sam's your guy!" Carol works with the new scientists to show them how to use chemical techniques to identify blood on dark surfaces. While the new scientists are proficient in DNA analysis, they had not been trained to *recognize and collect* possible DNA evidence. The *horizontal blood spatter on both sides* of Sam's shoes could not have been caused by vertical drops from his hands. The horizontal blood spatter was caused by blunt trauma to the victim while she was on the floor. The DNA lab quickly analyzes the horizontal blood spatter and confirms that the source of blood on the side of Sam's shoes is from victim Laura Lake. Presented with the new findings, Sam Livingston fully confesses to the killing of Laura Lake.

The combination of an experienced quality assurance manager, and new DNA technology ultimately solved the case. Sam's early alibi of an injury from yard work on the estate could not be eliminated, but it also could not be confirmed. Later analysis of the horizontal blood spatter on Sam's shoes puts him at the scene and excludes his alibi. The blood drop on the top of his shoe is blood from Sam's own injuries, but the injuries were not from clearing brush, they were caused when the victim, Laura Lake, fought for her life. The horizontal blood spatter on Sam's shoes was caused by the violent struggle on the floor. The blood spatter is at the same level as Sam's shoes. Laura Lake fought for her life and lost, but her struggle transferred evidence that resulted in the identification and prosecution of the defendant, Sam Livingston.

(continued)

CRIME SCENE

The police officers in charge of the Laura Lake homicide case, Detective Lieutenant Daniel Escobar and Detective Louis Muscato, have worked nonstop for one month trying to solve the case. They have gone over an endless number of hypotheses using multiple suspects, but always come back to Sam Livingston as the most probable person who could have committed this horrible crime. Sam was almost eliminated as a suspect several times, but the lieutenant's detective team could not confirm his alibi.

Lieutenant Escobar has worked with Carol on many cases when she was a serologist early in her career. He is not surprised that Carol broke the case with the recognition and subsequent DNA analysis of the horizontal blood spatter found upon Sam Livingston's shoes. In addition, the attorneys and the judge are all very impressed but not surprised with Carol's work. She had been a pivotal witness before the advent of DNA technology and now has used her experience to work with the new DNA scientists to solve this case.

The key to the Laura Lake homicide was the fact that the suspect's alibi could not be confirmed or excluded until the discovery of the horizontal blood spatter. The recognition of horizontal blood spatter followed by DNA analysis confirmed the presence of the victim's blood, thereby placing the suspect at the crime scene. The analysis of this evidence refuted the suspect's alibi that he was not at the scene.

CHAPTER 19

Becoming a Forensic Professional

The scientific advances noted throughout the book have created an explosion of interest in the forensic sciences as a profession. The paradox or *"CSI* effect" is that forensic science jobs are very demanding and quite different from those portrayed in the media. Increased demand has led some colleges to create "pseudoforensic" programs that take existing courses and give them forensic titles. These programs lack the substance required by the forensic community. As a result, graduates from substandard programs may lack appropriate skills and education and have difficulty finding employment in accredited labs.

Guidelines have been created to provide colleges and universities with standards for setting up academic programs of excellence. The National Institute of Justice (NIJ) in conjunction with West Virginia University put together the Technical Working Group on Education and Training in Forensic Science (TWGED). These scientists, educators, and practitioners developed the 2004 document entitled "Education and Training in Forensic Science: A Guide for Forensic Science Laboratories, Educational Institutions, and Students."

Subsequently, the American Academy of Forensic Science (AAFS) established the Forensic Education Programs Accreditation Commission (FEPAC). FEPAC's mission is "to maintain and to enhance the quality of forensic science education through a formal evaluation and recognition of college-level academic programs. The primary function of the Commission is to develop and to maintain standards and to administer an accreditation program that recognizes and distinguishes high quality undergraduate and graduate forensic science programs."

In 2003, FEPAC adopted the TWGED document as the national standard for all undergraduate and graduate programs. To date there are over 300 academic forensics programs in the United States; 14 have received FEPAC approval. FEPAC is not all-inclusive but rather a beginning set of standards for all forensic academic programs. Some extremely good forensic programs have not yet received FEPAC approval.

Differentiating between "pseudoforensic" and "highly competent forensic" can be established by investigating the program. Prospective students should ask basic questions such as the following:

- How long has the program been in existence? How many students have graduated?
- Are there forensic practitioners that are part of the faculty?
- Is there a forensic laboratory/agency associated with the existing forensic academic program?
- Does the program include internships or research projects? Are these assigned or is the student responsible for finding them?
- Is the university or college accredited by a body recognized by the U.S. Department of Education, i.e., the Middle States Commission on Higher Education?
- What are the facilities? Do students learn up-to-date theory? Do students practice using state-of-the-art technology?
- Does the program include a natural science core? Does the program require course work in the various forensic science disciplines?

Prospective students can arrange a personal visit to meet with the program director, faculty, and students. Ideally, the program is part of an accredited institution that is recognized by the U.S. Department of Education and has FEPAC approval, and, ideally, there are alumni who can be contacted and who can speak about their careers since graduating from the program. Full-time forensic scientists should take part in program instruction. These practitioners have knowledge in the most current forensic practices and theories and share their knowledge through lecture and laboratory course work. Ideally, the program collaborates with the forensic community to create, develop, and implement training. Partnerships with local law enforcement and other agencies provide training in the various disciplines in forensic science. An important distinction is that the ultimate goal of a forensic program is to produce scientists, not technicians.

An internship or an independent research project is required in many programs. There are a number of ways in which students can fulfill internship/research requirements. Students can complete a basic/applied research project or a comprehensive validation study. The students will take the knowledge and skills they obtained in their course work and apply them to a research project that is potentially applicable to forensic science and will be performed in a laboratory setting. After completion of the project, a detailed scientific report must be submitted for review and evaluation. In addition, many programs require students to present the project to their peers.

Students can arrange an internship in one of two ways: by finding a laboratory that they are interested in working in, or by asking the program director and/or faculty to help locate an appropriate laboratory facility in which the student can fulfill this requirement. Internships are paid or unpaid and are important in establishing a mentor relationship with a forensic professional. Many students also choose to volunteer in local laboratories to continue learning as well as to build ties with the forensic community.

A successful program will provide information about graduates from the program as well as contact information for recent graduates. Successful programs also have career placement and development centers. Career services may include help with résumés and cover letter reviews, mock interviews and networking, as well as helping with letters of recommendation. Students are also advised to take advantage of the extensive career services provided by the forensic community, such as the American Academy of Forensic Sciences, American Society of Crime Laboratory Directors, the Northeastern Association of Forensic Scientists, and other programs.

An excellent program will offer state-of-the-art technology such as DNA or serology. For example, students are trained on the most current equipment, software, and standard operating procedures currently used in forensic laboratories. Laboratories are often set up on campus to mirror laboratories at currently operating forensic facilities. Natural science courses are required, such as chemistry, biology, physics, and mathematics.

Excellent programs also have instruction in communication skills, both written and verbal. Programs should include course work in the law, ethics, and professional practices, evidence identification, collection and processing, quality assurance, and courtroom testimony. Much of this information can be covered in lecture, but a program that offers hands-on training is highly desirable. Eventually a forensic scientist is going to have to testify in court. Not only does she have to have an understanding of the natural sciences, but she must also have an understanding of the courtroom process, a familiarity with the other forensic disciplines (e.g., evidence identification, collecting, and processing), and must give her testimony in an unbiased, ethical manner that supports all quality assurance practices.

There are differences between undergraduate and graduate programs. A graduate program, such as a master's in science in forensic molecular biology, is for those students who are interested in becoming a technical leader, a supervisor, or a director of a smaller forensic laboratory. However, to apply for these supervisory level positions, students generally need at least three years of bench experience. Today, many laboratory director positions require a doctoral degree from an accredited university or college.

An undergraduate four-year program is very good for the forensic scientist who wants to be a nonsupervisory practitioner—a scientist who wants to work and be a valuable asset to a lab but not run it. These scientists will testify and perform all nonsupervisory bench work and laboratory support like validation studies, quality control, and quality assurance. Most undergraduate programs have an internship/research requirement like graduate school does. These internships provide additional bench work and analytical and interpretive skills necessary for work in the forensic field. In addition, an internship should require that all students present their results in a written scientific paper followed by an oral presentation. An internship is a great way to network with the forensic community and establish the possibility of a mentor relationship with local forensic professionals.

To find colleges and universities with the desired program, students can use the Internet. Specific regional forensic websites, such as the Northeastern Association of Forensic Scientists (NEAFS), and national websites, such as the American Academy of Forensic Sciences (AAFS) and the American Society of Crime Laboratory Directors (ASCLD), provide lists of programs. These websites list FEPAC-approved programs and also provide scholarship information. Privately run forensic websites, such as Reddy's, give listings of all of the academic programs, both graduate and undergraduate. These listings not only provide information on academic programs, but they give information on forensic science in general, plus employment opportunities. The information provided includes description of the program, the prerequisites for the program, the course requirements, grading policy, and internship requirements.

There are several ways for high school students to learn more about a career in forensic science. Many high schools have college credit forensic courses (for example, Syracuse University Project Advance [SUPA]). A four-year forensic degree would potentially lead to a nonadministrative forensic scientist position; alternatively, students obtain a bachelor's degree in a complimentary field and apply for the master's forensic degree with potential for a managerial position. Bachelor's degrees that are complimentary to the master's in forensics are those in biology, life sciences, chemistry, physics, criminal justice, and mathematics. Once the bachelor's degree is obtained, students then apply to the graduate program. High school students may also obtain internships at local forensic institutions, but these are noncredit, nonresearch-based volunteer internships. Internships at this level often include clerical and general nontechnical support for the forensic laboratory. However, these internships are extremely useful in allowing the student to get a general overview of the day-to-day operations in a forensic laboratory environment. These internships also provide networking, possibilities for letters of reference, and potential future employment opportunities.

Most graduates from a forensic program seeking employment as a forensic scientist in an accredited laboratory will have to undergo a background check. Depending on the agency or company, the background check may be quite extensive and include fingerprinting, a lie detector test, and drug screening. Most background checks take six months or more to complete.

As previously mentioned, a good program has a career placement office. Program directors and the school faculty are also important sources of employment opportunities. Websites such as Reddy's, the AAFS, and the ASCLD will have current listings posted. Word of mouth from past graduates as well as practitioners is key to finding new employment opportunities. Mentors from volunteer lab work internships will also be valuable sources in finding a job. Students should keep an updated curriculum vitae, have official transcripts available upon request, and obtain at least three letters of recommendation either from professors, internship advisors, the program director, or mentors.

Once hired, forget *CSI*—this is the real world! Crimes are not solved in 60 minutes, with time for commercials. A degree from a college or university provides a very solid foundation in the forensic sciences. Once hired by a forensic agency, however, new employees are required to successfully complete an intensive training program. The first six months to two years will involve additional training and competency testing. Upon successful completion of that training, forensic scientists are given more responsibilities and casework. Currently, most labs do a one-on-one training with new hires, which can take at least 12 to 18 months. During this period employees are expected to perform all standard operating procedures of the laboratory, learn basic usage and troubleshooting of all equipment, use of various software programs, proper documentation, chain of custody, quality assurance, and proper testimony procedures.

Recently, forensic laboratories have been using specialized training facilities to eliminate the one-on-one mentor system. Specialized training allows for small classes, intense, concise bench work, and a shorter time investment for training than the traditional one-on-one mentor system. Most newly hired forensic scientists going through specialized training programs will be required to spend 12 to 16 weeks at the training facility (i.e., University at Albany, Northeast Regional Forensic Institute *www.albany.edu/nerfi/dna*). However, an additional three months of training is also required back at the parent forensic laboratory. Once this training is complete, there are still continuous training opportunities that are required in most accredited forensic laboratories. Some forensic disciplines, such as DNA, require their forensic scientists to complete at least eight hours of continuing education each year. This requirement is usually completed through national meetings, regional meetings, and workforce development programs.

Other continuing education opportunities include certification programs provided by the American Board of Criminalistics (ABC). Passing the examinations provided by the ABC (e.g., FSAT) demonstrates a level of competency supported by the forensic community. Some of the examinations currently provided by the ABC include forensic biology, trace evidence, fire debris analysis, and drug chemistry. It is highly recommended that all new hires and senior-level scientists achieve these certifications and continue their education in the forensic sciences because the technology is changing rapidly every day.

Selected References

Associated Press. 2006. Lawyers of man convicted of 24 deaths ask for DNA tests. *USA Today* (11-29-06).

Bailey, F. L., and H. Aronson. 1971. *The Defense Never Rests.* New York: Signet.

Becker, W. S. 2006. In the crime lab. *The Industrial-Organizational Psychologist* 43 (4): 21–27.

Becker, W. S., and W. M. Dale. 2007. Critical human resource issues: Scientists under pressure. *Forensic Science Communications* 9 (2).

Becker, W. S., and W. M. Dale. 2003. Strategic human resource management in the forensic science laboratory. *Forensic Science Communications* 5 (4).

Becker, W. S., W. M. Dale, A. Lambert, and D. Magnus. 2005. Forensic lab directors' perceptions of staffing issues. *Journal of Forensic Sciences* 50 (5): 1255–1257.

Butler, J. M. 2005. *Forensic DNA Typing.* Amsterdam: Academic Press.

Chisum, W. J., and B. E. Turvey. 2000. Evidence dynamics: Locard's exchange principle and crime reconstruction. *Journal of Behavioral Profiling* 1 (1).

Conan Doyle, A. 1967. *The Annotated Sherlock Holmes,* ed. W. S. Baring-Gould. New York: Clarkson N. Potter.

Conners, B. F. *Tailspin: The Strange Call of Major Call.* Latham: British American Publishing.

Dale, W. M. 2004. The increase of forensic intellectual capital derived from a forensic advisory group: Measure intellectual capital and you can manage intellectual capital. Master's thesis, University at Albany, Albany, NY.

Dale, W. M., and W. S. Becker. 2005. Managing intellectual capital. *Forensic Science Communications* 7 (4).

Dale, W. M., and W. S. Becker. 2004. A case study of forensic scientist turnover. *Forensic Science Communications* 6 (4).

Dale, W. M., and W. S. Becker. 2003. Strategy for staffing forensic scientists. *Journal of Forensic Sciences* 48 (2): 465–466.

Dao, J. 2005. Lab's errors in '82 killing force review of Virginia DNA cases. *New York Times,* May 7.

DiMaio, D. J., and V. J. M. DiMaio. 1989. *Forensic Pathology.* New York: Elsevier.

DNA Advisory Board. 2000. Quality assurance standards for forensic DNA testing laboratories and for convicted offender DNA databasing laboratories. *Forensic Science Communications* 2 (3).

Fisher, B. A. 2003. Field needs adequate funding. National Forensic Science Commission. *Forensic Focus: Advancing the Forensic Science and Criminal Justice Communities.*

Giannelli, P. C. 2003. Crime labs need improvement. *Issues in Science and Technology,* 20, 1, 55–58.

Goodwin, M., and C. DeMare. 2007. No release for baby killer. *Albany Times-Union,* Albany, NY, March 30.

Haapanen, R. A. 1998. *Selective Incapacitation and the Serious Offender: A Longitudinal Study of Criminal Career Patterns.* Sacramento, CA: California Department of the Youth Authority.

Halbfinger, D. M. 2002. Retracing a trail: Sniper clue sat for weeks in crime lab in Alabama. *New York Times,* October 26.

Helpern, M., and B. Knight. 1977. *Autopsy: The Memoirs of Milton Helpern, The World's Greatest Medical Detective.* New York: St. Martin's Press.

Hornfeldt, C. S., Lothridge, K. and Upshaw Downs, J. C. 2002. Forensic Science Update: Gamma-hydroxybutrate (GHB). *Forensic Science Communications, 4,* 1.

International Laboratory Accreditation Cooperation (ILAC). 2001. *Guidance for Accreditation to ISO/IEC 17025.*

International Laboratory Accreditation Cooperation (ILAC). 2002. *Guidelines for Forensic Science Laboratories.*

Jeffreys, A. J. 2005. Genetic fingerprinting. *Nature Medicine* 11 (10): 1035–1039.

Jeffreys, A. J., J. F. Brookfield, and R. Semeonoff. 1985. Positive identification of an immigration test-case using human DNA fingerprints. *Nature* 317 (6040): 818–819.

Jeffreys, A. J., V. Wilson, and S. L. Thein. 1985. Individual-specific "fingerprints" of human DNA. *Nature* 316 (6023): 76–79.

Kanable, R. 2005. Modern forensic science today and tomorrow: An interview with Dr. Henry Lee. *Law Enforcement Technology* 32 (7).

Koussiafes, P. M. 2004. Public forensic laboratory budget issues. *Forensic Science Communication* 6 (3).

Lucas, D. M. 1989. The ethical responsibilities of the forensic scientist: Exploring the limits. *Journal of Forensic Sciences* 34:719–729.

National Institute of Justice. 2003. DNA in "minor" crimes yields major benefits in public safety. Office of Justice Programs.

O'Hara, C. E., and J. W. Osterburg. 1949. *An Introduction to Criminalistics: The Application of the Physical Sciences to the Detection of Crime.* New York: MacMillan.

Page, K. 2003. Reformers aim to shake up British system. *Science* 301 (5633): 579.

Peterson, J. L. 1989. Symposium: Ethical conflicts in the forensic sciences. *Journal of Forensic Sciences* 34 (3): 717–718.

Peterson, J. L., D. Crim, J. E. Murdock, and M. Crim. 1989. Forensic science ethics: Developing an integrated system of support and enforcement. *Journal of Forensic Sciences* 34 (3): 749–762.

Peterson, J. L., and M. J. Hickman. 2005. Census of publicly funded forensic crime laboratories. *Bureau of Justice Statistics Bulletin*, February.

Plumin, R., and J. Crabbe. 2000. DNA. *Psychological Bulletin* 126 (6): 806–828.

Preston, J. 2005. For '73 rape victim, DNA revives horror, too. *New York Times*, November 3.

Pyrek, K. M. 2007. *Forensic Science Under Siege.* Amsterdam: Academic Press.

Rudin, N., and K. Inman. 2001. *Principles and Practice of Forensic Science: The Profession of Forensic Science.* Boca Raton, FL: CRC Press.

Scientific Working Group on DNA Analysis Methods (SWGDAM). 2000. Short tandem repeat (STR) interpretation guidelines. *Forensic Science Communications* 2 (3).

Scientific Working Group on DNA Analysis Methods (SWGDAM). 2003. Bylaws of the Scientific Working Group on DNA Analysis Methods. *Forensic Science Communications* 5 (2).

Scientific Working Group on DNA Analysis Methods (SWGDAM). 2004. Revised Validation Guidelines. *Forensic Science Communications* 6 (3).

Sewell, J. D. 2000. Identifying and mitigating stress among forensic laboratory managers. *Forensic Science Communications* 2 (2).

Simon, L. M. J. 1997. Do criminal offenders specialize in crime types? *Applied and Preventive Psychology* 6:35–53.

Spitz, W. U., and R. S. Fisher. 1993. *Medicolegal Investigation of Death*, 3rd Edition. Springfield, IL: Charles C. Thomas.

Technical Analysis Group on DNA Analysis Methods. 1989. Guidelines for a quality assurance program for DNA restriction fragment length polymorphism analysis. *Crime Laboratory Digest* 16 (2).

Technical Analysis Group on DNA Analysis Methods and California Association of Criminalistics Ad Hoc Committee on DNA Quality Assurance. 1991. Guidelines for a quality assurance program for DNA analysis. *Crime Laboratory Digest* 18 (2).

Technical Analysis Group on DNA Analysis Methods. 1995. Guidelines for a quality assurance program for DNA analysis. *Crime Laboratory Digest* 22 (2).

Von Glinow, M. A.Y. 1988. *The New Professionals: Managing Today's High-Tech Employees.* Cambridge, MA: Ballinger.

Walsh, S. J. 2005. Legal perceptions of forensic DNA profiling part I: A review of the legal literature. *Forensic Science International* 155:51–60.

Colleges and Universities[1]

Programs accredited by the AAFS-FEPAC:

Albany State University
Bachelor of Science Degree in Forensic Science
504 College Drive
Albany, GA 31705
www.asurams.edu/forensicscience
(229) 430-4864

Charles O. Ochie Sr., Ph.D. "Ogbuefi"
Director, Forensic Science Program
charles.ochie@asurams.edu

Arcadia University
Master of Science Degree Program in Forensic Science
450 South Easton Road
Glenside, PA 19038
www.arcadia.edu
(267) 620-4140

Lawrence A. Presley, M.S., M.A., D-ABC
Director, Forensic Science Program
presley@arcadia.edu

---

1. Source: *www.AAFS.org*

Cedar Crest College

Bachelor of Science Degree Program in Chemistry, Biochemistry, Biology,
and Genetic Engineering with a concentration in Forensic Science
Department of Chemistry
100 College Drive
Allentown, PA 18104-6196
www.cedarcrest.edu
(610) 606-4666, ext. 3567

Lawrence Quarino, Ph.D.
laquarin@cedarcrest.edu

Eastern Kentucky University

Bachelor of Science Degree Program in Forensic Science
Forensic Science Program
521 Lancaster Avenue
Richmond, KY 40475-3102
www.chemistry.eku.edu/FORSCI
(859) 622-2908

Diane E. Vance, Ph.D.
diane.vance@eku.edu

Florida International University

Certificate Programs in conjunction with the Bachelor of Science in a
natural science such as Chemistry or Biology
Department of Chemistry
Miami, FL 33199
www.fiu.edu/ ~ ifri
(305) 348-6656

Alberto J. Sabucedo, Ph.D.
sabucedo@fiu.edu

Florida International University

Master of Science Degree Program in Forensic Science
Department of Chemistry
Miami, FL 33199
www.fiu.edu/ ~ ifri

Bruce R. McCord, Ph.D.
mccordb@fiu.edu

Marshall University

Master of Science Degree Program in Forensic Science
Forensic Science Center
1401 Forensic Science Drive
Huntington, WV 25701
forensics.marshall.edu/MUFSC_Homepage.htm
(304) 690-GENE (4363)

Terry W. Fenger, Ph.D.
fenger@marshall.edu

Metropolitan State College of Denver

Bachelor of Science Degree Program in Chemistry with a concentration
   in Criminalistics
Department of Chemistry
PO Box 173362
Campus Box 52
Denver, CO 80217-3362
www.mscd.edu
(303) 556-2610

Charles G. Tindall Jr., Ph.D.
tindallc@mscd.edu

Michigan State University

Master of Science Degree Program
(Biology and Chemistry tracks)
560A Baker Hall
East Lansing, MI 48824-1118
www.forensic.msu.edu
(517) 353-7133

Dr. David Foran
forsci@msu.edu

University of Mississippi

Bachelor of Science Degree in Forensic Chemistry
322 Coulter Hall
University, MS 38677
www.olemiss.edu/depts/chemistry/undergraduate/bs_forensic.php
(662) 915-5143

Murrell Godfrey, Ph.D.
Director, Forensic Chemistry Program
mgodfrey@olemiss.edu

Ohio University

Bachelor of Science Degree in Forensic Chemistry
Department of Chemistry & Biochemistry
Clippinger Laboratory
Athens, OH 45701-2979
www.chem.ohiou.edu/undergraduate/forensic.html
(740) 517-8458

Dr. Peter de B. Harrington
peter.harrington@ohio.edu

University at Albany
Master of Science Degree in Forensic Molecular Biology
1400 Washington Avenue
Albany, NY 12222
www.albany.edu/biology/forensics
(518) 442-4300

Donald D. Orokos, Ph.D.
Director, Forensic Molecular Biology Program
orokos@albany.edu

Virginia Commonwealth University
Bachelor of Science Degree in Forensic Science and Master of Science
  Degree in Forensic Science
College of Humanities & Sciences
1000 West Franklin Street
PO Box 843079
Richmond, VA 23284-3079
www.has.vcu.edu/forensics
(804) 828-8420
Fax: (804) 828-4983

Dr. William B. Eggleston
weggles@saturn.vcu.edu

West Chester University
Bachelor of Science Degree Program in Forensic and Toxicological
  Chemistry
Department of Chemistry
West Chester, PA 19383
www.wcupa.edu
(610) 436-2780

Blaise F. Frost, Ph.D.
bfrost@wcupa.edu

West Virginia University

Bachelor of Science Degree—Forensic and Investigative Science Program

Forensic and Analytical Chemistry

217 Clark Hall

PO Box 6045

Morgantown, WV 26506

www.wvu.edu/ ~ forensic

(304) 293-3435, ext. 6436

Fax: (304) 293-4904

Dr. Suzanne Bell

suzanne.bell@mailwvu.edu

More Resources in the Forensic Sciences

American Academy of Forensic Sciences (AAFS)
www.aafs.org

American Board of Forensic Toxicology (ABFT)
www.abft.org

American Society of Crime Laboratory Directors (ASCLD)
www.ascld.org

American Society of Crime Laboratory Directors/Laboratory Accreditation Board (ASCLD/LAB)
www.ascld-lab.org

American Society of Questioned Document Examiners (ASQDE)
www.asqde.org

California Association of Criminalistics (CAC)
www.cacnews.org

Canadian Society of Forensic Science (CSFS)
www.csfs.ca/index.htm

The Criminal Justice Information System (CJIS)
www.fbi.gov/hq/cjisd/cjis.htm

Federal Bureau of Investigation (FBI)
www.fbi.gov

Innocence Project
www.innocenceproject.com

International Association for Identification (IAI)
www.theiai.org

International Association of Forensic Nurses (IAFN)
www.forensicnurse.org

Mid-Atlantic Association of Forensic Scientists (MAAFS)
www.maafs.org

National Association of Medical Examiners (NAME)
www.thename.org

National Center for Forensic Science (NCFS)
www.ncfs.org

National District Attorneys Association (NDAA)
www.ndaa-apri.org

National Forensic Science Technology Center (NFSTC)
www.nfstc.org/index.htm

Reddy's Forensic Page
www.forensicpage.com

Society of Forensic Toxicologists (SOFT)
www.soft-tox.org

Southern Association of Forensic Scientists (SAFS)
www.southernforensic.org

The International Association of Forensic Toxicologists (TIAFT)
www.tiaft.org

U.S. Census
www.us.census.gov

Zeno's Forensic Site
www.forensic.to/forensic.html

Forensic Science Technician Job Analysis[1]

Summary report for forensic science technicians: Collect, identify, classify, and analyze physical evidence related to criminal investigations. Perform tests on weapons or substances, such as fiber, hair, and tissue to determine significance to investigation. May testify as expert witnesses on evidence or crime laboratory techniques. May serve as specialists in area of expertise, such as ballistics, fingerprinting, handwriting, or biochemistry.

Sample of reported job titles: Criminalist, Crime Scene Technician, Crime Scene Investigator, Evidence Technician, Crime Scene Analyst, Detective—Crime Scene Investigations, Forensic Scientist, Latent Fingerprint Examiner

Tasks

- Testify in court about investigative and analytical methods and findings
- Keep records and prepare reports detailing findings, investigative methods, and laboratory techniques
- Interpret laboratory findings and test results to identify and classify substances, materials, and other evidence collected at crime scenes
- Operate and maintain laboratory equipment and apparatus
- Prepare solutions, reagents, and sample formulations needed for laboratory work

---

1. Source: *online.onetcenter.org/link/summary/19-4092.00*

- Collect evidence from crime scenes, storing it in conditions that preserve its integrity
- Identify and quantify drugs and poisons found in biological fluids and tissues, in foods, and at crime scenes
- Reconstruct crime scenes to determine relationships among pieces of evidence
- Collect impressions of dust from surfaces to obtain and identify fingerprints
- Analyze gunshot residue and bullet paths to determine how shootings occurred

Knowledge

Chemistry—Knowledge of the chemical composition, structure, and properties of substances and of the chemical processes and transformations that they undergo. This includes uses of chemicals and their interactions, danger signs, production techniques, and disposal methods.

Law and Government—Knowledge of laws, legal codes, court procedures, precedents, government regulations, executive orders, agency rules, and the democratic political process.

English Language—Knowledge of the structure and content of the English language including the meaning and spelling of words, rules of composition, and grammar.

Customer and Personal Service—Knowledge of principles and processes for providing customer and personal services. This includes customer needs assessment, meeting quality standards for services, and evaluation of customer satisfaction.

Public Safety and Security—Knowledge of relevant equipment, policies, procedures, and strategies to promote effective local, state, or national security operations for the protection of people, data, property, and institutions.

Skills

Science—Using scientific rules and methods to solve problems.

Speaking—Talking to others to convey information effectively.

Quality Control Analysis—Conducting tests and inspections of products, services, or processes to evaluate quality or performance.

Reading Comprehension—Understanding written sentences and paragraphs in work-related documents.

Critical Thinking—Using logic and reasoning to identify the strengths and weaknesses of alternative solutions, conclusions, or approaches to problems.

Active Listening—Giving full attention to what other people are saying, taking time to understand the points being made, asking questions as appropriate, and not interrupting at inappropriate times.

Writing—Communicating effectively in writing as appropriate for the needs of the audience.

Active Learning—Understanding the implications of new information for both current and future problem solving and decision making.

Equipment Selection—Determining the kind of tools and equipment needed to do a job.

Coordination—Adjusting actions in relation to others' actions.

Abilities

Inductive Reasoning—The ability to combine pieces of information to form general rules or conclusions (includes finding a relationship among seemingly unrelated events).

Near Vision—The ability to see details at close range (within a few feet of the observer).

Oral Expression—The ability to communicate information and ideas through speaking so others will understand.

Oral Comprehension—The ability to listen to and understand information and ideas presented through spoken words and sentences.

Speech Clarity—The ability to speak clearly so others can understand you.

Deductive Reasoning—The ability to apply general rules to specific problems to produce answers that make sense.

Information Ordering—The ability to arrange things or actions in a certain order or pattern according to a specific rule or set of rules (e.g., patterns of numbers, letters, words, pictures, mathematical operations).

Written Expression—The ability to communicate information and ideas in writing so others will understand.

Problem Sensitivity—The ability to tell when something is wrong or is likely to go wrong. It does not involve solving the problem, only recognizing there is a problem.

Category Flexibility—The ability to generate or use different sets of rules for combining or grouping things in different ways.

ILAC Guidelines for Forensic Science Laboratories and International Standard ISO/IEC 17025

Accreditation and education are the keys to ensuring quality in forensic science. The American Society of Crime Laboratory Directors (ASCLD) developed its own accreditation program for forensic laboratories. ASCLD was formed in 1973 with the assistance of the FBI laboratory; its mission is to promote forensic excellence through leadership and innovation. ASCLD formed the American Society of Crime Laboratory Directors/Laboratory Accreditation Board (ASCLD/LAB) in 1982. ASCLD/LAB developed its own team of auditors to provide external review of all laboratory policies and procedures. Several states, including New York, Oklahoma, and Texas, have legislatively mandated compliance with the ASCLD/LAB program. The ASCLD/LAB program now embraces the ISO/IEC 17025:2005 industry standard to further enhance quality in an international context. In 1996, ASCLD formed the National Forensic Science Technology Center (NFSTC) to provide training and professional development programs for the forensic community. Two documents—the ILAC G19 and the introduction to ISO/IEC 17025:2005—are provided here. More information about these professional organizations can be found at the following websites:

www.ascld.org
www.ascld-lab.org
www.nfstc.org

GUIDELINES FOR FORENSIC SCIENCE LABORATORIES
ILAC-G19:2002

©Copyright ILAC 2002

ILAC encourages the authorised reproduction of its publications, or parts thereof, by organisations wishing to use such material for areas related to education, standardisation, accreditation, good laboratory practice or other purposes relevant to ILAC's area of expertise or endeavour.

Organisations seeking permission to reproduce material from ILAC publications must contact the ILAC Chair or Secretariat in writing or via electronic means such as email.

The request for permission should clearly detail

1) the ILAC publication, or part thereof, for which permission is sought;
2) where the reproduced material will appear and what it will be used for;
3) whether the document containing the ILAC material will be distributed commercially, where it will be distributed or sold, and what quantities will be involved;
4) any other background information that may assist ILAC to grant permission.

ILAC reserves the right to refuse permission without disclosing the reasons for such refusal. The document in which the reproduced material appears must contain a statement acknowledging ILAC's contribution to the document.

ILAC's permission to reproduce its material only extends as far as detailed in the original request. Any variation to the stated use of the ILAC material must be notified in advance in writing to ILAC for additional permission.

ILAC shall not be held liable for any use of its material in another document.

Any breach of the above permission to reproduce or any unauthorised use of ILAC material is strictly prohibited and may result in legal action.

To obtain permission or for further assistance, please contact:

The ILAC Secretariat,
c/- NATA,
7 Leeds Street,
Rhodes, NSW, Australia, 2138,
Fax: + 61 2 9743 5311,
Email: *ilac@nata.asn.au*

Preamble

The general requirements for the competence of testing and calibration laboratories are described in ISO/IEC 17025. These requirements are designed to apply to all types of calibration and objective testing and therefore need to be interpreted with respect to the type of calibration and testing concerned and the techniques involved.

This document does not re-state all the provisions of ISO/IEC 17025 and laboratories are reminded of the need to comply with all of the relevant criteria detailed in ISO/IEC 17025. The clause numbers in this document follow those of ISO/ IEC 17025 but since not all clauses require interpretation, the numbering may not be continuous.

This document may also be used by accreditation bodies to provide appropriate criteria for the assessment and accreditation of laboratories providing forensic services.

Laboratories are also reminded of the need to comply with any relevant statutory or legislative requirements.

Purpose

This document is intended to provide guidance for laboratories involved in forensic analysis and examination by providing application of ISO/IEC 17025.

Authorship

This document has been produced in consultation with Working Group 4 of the ILAC Technical Accreditation Issues Committee, and approved for publication by the ILAC General Assembly in 2001.

1. SCOPE

Forensic science refers to the examination of scenes of crime, recovery of evidence, laboratory examinations, interpretation of findings and presentation of the conclusions reached for intelligence purposes or for use in court. The activities range from instrumental analysis with unequivocal results, such as blood alcohol determination and glass refractive index measurement, to the investigation of suspicious fires and vehicle accidents, to comparison work such as handwriting and toolmark examination, which is largely subjective in nature but which, with training, can produce consistent outcomes between different forensic scientists.

1.1 Forensic science work involves the examination of a wide range of items and substances. The following list describes the activities that may be encountered in a forensic laboratory. This does not, however, preclude other activities being undertaken in a forensic laboratory.

Controlled Substances
- Controlled pharmaceutical and illicit drugs
- Related chemicals and paraphernalia
- Botanical material

Toxicology
- Pharmaceutical products
- Poisons
- Alcohol

Hairs, Blood, Body Fluids and Tissues
- Serology
- DNA profiling

Trace Evidence
- Fire debris
- Pyrotechnic devices
- Glass
- Pain
- Metals and alloys
- Fibres and hairs
- Adhesives
- Oils and greases
- Lachrymatory chemicals
- Fertilisers
- Acids
- Food

- Feedingstuffs and ancillary items
- Components of technical or household appliances
- Botanical material (excluding controlled substances)
- Hydrocarbon fuels
- Explosives and explosion debris
- Light filaments
- Vehicle components
- Firearm discharge residues
- Clothing/garments
- Dyes and pigments
- Cosmetics
- Soils
- Corrosives
- Alkalis
- Lubricants and spermicidal agents
- Electrical devices and components
- Manufacturers marks (incl serial number restoration)

Firearms and Ballistics
- Firearms
- Bullets and cartridges

Handwriting and Document Examination
- Handwriting
- Paper
- Rubber stamps
- Security marks
- Printers and other printed objects
- Inks and printing materials
- Copiers and copied material
- Indentations
- Typewriters and typewritten material

Fingerprints
- Fingerprints
- Footprints
- Palmprints

Marks and Impressions
- Toolmarks

- Shoe prints
- Glove marks
- Toolmarks and impressions
- Tyre prints
- Fabric prints
- Non-friction ridge body prints

Audio, Video and Computer Analysis
- Audiotape recordings
- Language samples
- Image enhancement
- Facial mapping
- Speech samples
- Computers (hardware and software)
- Videogrammetry
- Recovery of information

Accident Investigation
- Tachograph charts
- Component failures
- Speed calculations
- Car immobiliser systems
- Trace evidence
- Unsafe loads
- Electrical failures

Scene Investigation
- Crime scene investigation
- Computer simulations
- Fire investigation
- Evidence recovery
- Photography
- Blood splash pattern interpretation

Forensic pathology, Entomology, Odontology

1.2 The techniques adopted in the analysis and examination of forensic material cover a broad range from visual examination to sophisticated instrumental procedures. Techniques which are employed include but are not limited to:

- Chemical colour tests
- Chemiluminescence
- Chromatography
- Atomic absorption and emission spectrometry
- Ultraviolet, infrared and visible spectrophotometry
- Optical and electron microscopy
- Serology
- Electrophoresis
- Metallurgy
- Autoradiography
- DNA analysis
- Mass spectrometry
- Nuclear magnetic resonance spectroscopy
- Physical measurements eg weight, volume, length, density, refractive index
- X-ray analysis
- Immunoassay
- Visual inspections
- Computer simulations

It is anticipated that the majority of the work carried out in forensic science laboratories will be capable of satisfying the definition of an objective test, although in some instances a different emphasis may be placed on the particular aspect of 'control' required. The level of training and experience for staff involved in the work will be dependent on the nature of the examination or test.

2. REFERENCES

ISO/IEC 17025:1999, *General requirements for the competence of testing and calibration laboratories.*

ISO/IEC Guide 2, *General terms and their definitions concerning standardisation and related activities.*

ISO Guide 30:1992, *Terms and definitions used in connection with reference materials.*

ILAC-P10: 2002, *ILAC Policy on Traceability of Measurement Results*

ILAC-G2: 1994, *Traceability of measurements*

3.   **TERMS AND DEFINITIONS**

For the purposes of the Guide, the relevant terms and definitions given in ISO/IEC Guide 2 apply.

Objective Test

A test which having been documented and validated is under control so that it can be demonstrated that all appropriately trained staff will obtain the same results within defined limits. These defined limits relate to expressions of degrees of probability as well as numerical values.

Objective tests will be controlled by:

- documentation of the test
- validation of the test
- training and authorisation of staff
- maintenance of equipment

and where appropriate by;

- calibration of equipment
- use of appropriate reference materials
- provision of guidance for interpretation
- checking of results
- testing of staff proficiency
- recording of equipment/test performance

Visual inspection, qualitative examinations and computer simulations are included in the definition of objective test.

Reference Collection

A collection of stable materials, substances, objects or artefacts of known properties or origin that may be used in the determination of the properties or origins of unknown items.

Court Statement

A written report of the results and interpretations of forensic tests/examinations submitted to court. Such reports may be in a format prescribed in legislation.

4.   MANAGEMENT REQUIREMENTS

4.12   Control of Records

4.12.2.1 a) The forensic science laboratory should have documented procedures to ensure that it maintains a coordinated record relating to each case under investigation. The information that is to be included in case records should be documented and may include records of telephone conversations, evidence receipts, descriptions of evidence packaging and seals, subpoenas, records of observations and test/examination results, reference to procedures used, diagrams, print-outs, autoradiographs, photographs, etc. In general, the records required to support conclusions should be such that in the absence of the analyst/examiner, another competent analyst/examiner could evaluate what had been performed and interpret the data.

b) Where instrumental analyses are conducted, operating parameters should be recorded.

c) Where appropriate, observations or test results should be preserved by photography or electronic scanning (eg electrophoretic runs, physical matches). Photocopies, tracings or hand-drawn facsimiles may also be suitable (eg thin-layer chromatography results, questioned documents).

d) When a test result or observation is rejected, the reason(s) should be recorded.

e) Calculations and data transfers which do not form part of a validated electronic process should be checked, preferably by a second person. The case record should include an indication that such checks have been carried out and by whom.

f) Each page of every document in the case record should be traceable to the analyst/examiner and where appropriate, to a uniquely identified case or exhibit. It should be clear from the case record who has performed all stages of the analysis/examination and when each stage of the analysis/examination was performed (eg relevant date(s)).

g) Laboratory generated examination records should be paginated using a page numbering system which indicates the total number of pages.

h) The laboratory should have documented policies and procedures for the review of case records, including test reports.

Where independent checks on critical findings are carried out by other authorised personnel, the records should indicate that each critical finding has been checked and agreed and by whom the checks were performed. This may be indicated in a number of ways including entries against each finding, entry on a summary of findings or a statement to this effect in the records.

5. TECHNICAL REQUIREMENTS

5.2 Personnel

5.2.1 The laboratory should have a defined policy that ensures that all staff working in the laboratory are competent to perform the work required. The term 'competent' implies possessing the requisite knowledge, skills and abilities to perform the job. The laboratory's policy should also include procedures for retraining and maintenance of skills and expertise.

Where test or technique specific training is given, acceptance criteria should be assigned eg observation of the relevant tests or analyses by an experienced officer, satisfactory performance in the analysis of quality control/quality assurance samples, correlation of results with those obtained by other trained staff. Where necessary, training programs should also include training in the presentation of evidence in court.

5.2.5 A laboratory should have clear statements of the competencies required for all jobs and records should be maintained to demonstrate that all staff are competent for the jobs they are asked to carry out.

Each laboratory or section should maintain an up-to-date record of the training that each member of staff has received. These records should include academic and professional qualifications, external or internal courses attended and relevant training (and retraining, where necessary) received whilst working in the laboratory.

Records should be sufficiently detailed to provide evidence that staff performing particular tasks have been properly trained and that their subsequent ability to perform these tests has been formally assessed.

5.3   Accommodation and Environmental Conditions

5.3.3   Special care is needed in forensic testing laboratories involved in the analysis or determination of trace levels of materials, including DNA. Physical separation of high-level and low-level work is required. Where special areas are set aside for this type of work, access to these areas should be restricted and the work undertaken carefully controlled. Appropriate records should be kept to demonstrate this control. It may also be necessary to carry out 'environmental monitoring' of equipment, work areas, clothing and consumables.

5.3.4   a) Access to the operational area of the laboratory should be controllable and limited. Visitors should not have unrestricted access to the operational areas of the laboratory. A record should be retained of all visitors to the operational areas of the laboratory.

b) Evidence storage areas should be secure to prevent theft or interference and there should be limited, controlled access. The storage conditions should be such as to prevent loss, deterioration and contamination and to maintain the integrity and identity of the evidence. This applies both before and after examinations have been performed.

5.4   Test and calibration methods and method validation

5.4.1   All methods should be fully documented including procedures for quality control, and, where appropriate, the use of reference materials.

5.4.2   a) All technical procedures used by a forensic science laboratory should be fully validated before being used on casework.

b) Where a laboratory introduces a new (validated) method, it should first demonstrate the reliability of the procedure in-house against any documented performance characteristics of that procedure. Records of performance verification should be maintained for future reference.

c) Laboratories should institute a procedure to identify infrequently performed tests or analyses. For these tests or analyses, there are two methods of demonstrating competence, either of which would be equally valid. These are:

i. regular analysis of control samples and use of control charts even when casework samples are not being analysed; or

ii. reverification before the test or analysis in question is performed on a casework sample involving at least the use of an appropriate reference material, followed by replicate testing or analysis of the real sample.

d) The quality of standard materials and reagents should be adequate for the procedure used. Lot/batch numbers of standard materials and critical reagents should be recorded. All critical reagents should be tested for their reliability.

Standard materials and reagents should be labelled with:

- name;
- concentration, where appropriate,
- preparation date and or expiry date;
- identity of preparer;
- storage conditions, if relevant;
- hazard warning, where necessary.

5.4.5.1 All technical procedures used by a forensic science laboratory must be fully validated before being used on casework.

Methods may be validated by comparison with other established methods using certified reference materials (where available) or materials of known characteristics. In validating test methods, the following issues (among others) may need to be determined, as appropriate:

- matrix effects
- interferences
- sample homogeneity
- concentration ranges
- specificity
- stability of measured compounds

- linearity range
- population distribution
- precision
- measurement uncertainty

Validation studies can be conducted by the scientific community (as in the case of standard or published methods) or by the forensic science laboratory itself (as in the case of methods developed inhouse or where significant modifications are made to previously validated methods).

5.5   Equipment

5.5.2   As part of a quality system, all laboratories are required to operate a program for the maintenance and calibration of equipment used in the laboratory. The equipment used in a forensic science laboratory is diverse and will range across a number of different scientific and technical disciplines.

a) General service equipment not directly used for making measurements (e.g. hot plates, stirrers, non-volumetric glassware, cameras, refrigerators, thermal cyclers).

Such equipment will typically be maintained by visual examination, safety checks and cleaning as necessary. Calibrations or performance checks will only be necessary where the equipment setting can significantly affect the test or analytical result (eg temperature of a muffle furnace or constant temperature bath).

b) Microscopes including attachments

Microscopes should be cleaned and serviced periodically. Steps should be taken to ensure that microscopes are properly set up for use and are used only by competent staff. Where microscopes are used for measurement the guidance given in paragraph d) applies.

c) Volumetric equipment

Volumetric equipment will typically be maintained by visual examination and cleaning but calibration and performance checks will need to be carried out before initial use and at intervals depending on the type and frequency of use.

d) Measuring instruments—thermometers, balances, densitometers, chromatographs, spectrometers and spectrophotometers, refractometers, autoanalysers, DNA sequencers

Correct use combined with periodic servicing, cleaning and calibration will not necessarily ensure that a measuring instrument or detection system is performing adequately. Therefore, where appropriate, periodic performance checks shall be carried out and predetermined limits of acceptability shall be assigned. The frequency of such performance checks should be determined by need, type and previous performance of the equipment.

It is often possible to build performance checks or system suitability checks into test methods (eg chromatographic systems, measurement of glass refractive index). These checks should be documented and should be satisfactorily completed before the equipment is used or before results are accepted.

e) Computers and data processors

5.6   Measurement traceability

5.6.1   Individual calibration programs should be established depending on the specific requirements of the testing or analytical work being carried out. It will normally be necessary to check instrument calibration after any shut down, whether deliberate or otherwise, and following service or other substantial maintenance. In general, calibration intervals should not be less stringent than manufacturers' recommendations.

5.6.2.2.2 For many types of analysis, 'calibration' may be carried out using synthetic standards containing the analytes under test, prepared within the laboratory from chemicals of known purity and composition, or matrix matched standards. Alternatively, 'standard' solutions may be purchased. Many chemicals can be purchased with manufacturer's statements or certificates. Wherever possible, laboratories should obtain supplies of chemical standards from competent suppliers.

5.6.3.2 Reference collections of data or items/materials encountered in casework which are maintained for identification, comparison or interpretation purposes (eg mass spectra, motor vehicle paints or headlamp lenses, drug samples, typewriter printstyles, wood fragments, bullets, cartridges, DNA profiles, frequency databases) should be fully documented, uniquely identified and properly controlled.

5.7 Sampling

5.7.1 Selection, recovery, prioritisation and sampling of materials from submitted test items and from scenes of crime are important parts of the forensic process. In the area of forensic science emphasis is placed on the competence of the scientist and the training of staff in these activities is therefore of prime importance. Laboratories should ensure that there are documented procedures and training programs to cover this aspect of their work and that detailed competency/training records are kept for all staff involved.

5.8 Handling of test and calibration items

5.8.1 For legal purposes, forensic science laboratories should be able to demonstrate that the items/samples examined and reported on were those submitted to the laboratory. A 'chain of custody' record should be maintained from the receipt of items/samples which details each person who takes possession of an item or alternatively the location of that item (eg if in storage).

5.8.4 There should be documented procedures which describe the measures taken to secure exhibits in the process of being examined which must be left unattended.

5.9 Assuring the quality of test and calibration results

5.9.1 a) Analytical performance should be monitored by operating quality control schemes which are appropriate to the type and frequency of testing undertaken by a laboratory. The range of quality control activities available to laboratories includes the use of:

- reference collections;
- certified reference materials and internally generated reference materials;
- statistical tables;

- positive and negative controls;
- control charts;
- replicate testing;
- alternative methods;
- repeat testing;
- spiked samples, standard additions and internal standards;
- independent checks (verification) by other authorised personnel.

Depending on the particular test being performed, the laboratory may make use of one or several of these examples to demonstrate that the test or examination is 'under control'.

The quality control procedures necessary in any particular area of work should be determined by the laboratory responsible for the work, based on best professional practice. The procedures should be documented and records should be retained to show that all appropriate QC measures have been taken, that all QC results are acceptable or, if not, that remedial action has been taken.

b) An effective means for a forensic science laboratory to monitor its performance, both against its own requirements and against the performance of peer laboratories, is to take part in proficiency testing programs. When participating in proficiency testing programs, the laboratory's own documented test procedures should be used. Performance in the programs should be reviewed regularly and where necessary, corrective action should be taken.

Proficiency testing records should include:

- full details of the analyses/examinations undertaken and the results and conclusions obtained;
- an indication that performance has been reviewed;
- details of the corrective action undertaken, where necessary.

c) The laboratory should have and follow a documented procedure whereby the testimony of each examiner is monitored on a regular basis. The evaluation should include appearance, performance and effectiveness of presentation. The monitoring procedure should also prescribe the remedial action that is to be taken should the evaluation be less than satisfactory.

5.10   Reporting the results

5.10.2   It is accepted that forensic science laboratories may not be able to include all of the items in 'Court Statements' that are detailed in sub-clause 5.10 of ISO/IEC 17025 as the format of these documents is prescribed in legislation. Forensic science laboratories may therefore elect to adopt one or more of the following means of meeting these requirements.

  - the preparation of a test report which includes all of the information required by ISO/IEC 17025;
  - the preparation of an annex to the Court Statement which includes any additional information required by ISO/ IEC 17025;
  - ensuring that the case record relating to a specific investigation contains all the relevant information required by ISO/ IEC 17025.

Annex: Bibliography

ISO/IEC Application Document, Supplementary Requirements for Accreditation in the Field of Forensic Science: 2000 version 1, National Association of Testing Authorities, Australia (NATA).

Accreditation for Forensic Analysis and Examination, NIS 46, Edition 2, December 1994, United Kingdom Accreditation Service (UKAS).

American Society of Crime Laboratory Directors – *Laboratory Accreditation Board Manual,* 1999

NIS 96, *Accreditation for Suppliers to the UK National DNA Database,* March 1997, United Kingdom Accreditation Service (UKAS).

CAN-P-1578, *Guidelines for the Accreditation of Forensic Testing Laboratories,* 2nd Edition, November 1998, Standards Council of Canada (SCC).

Specific Criteria for Forensic Analysis, Raad voor Accreditatie (RVA), October 1993.

Reference number
ISO/IEC 17025:2005(E)
©ISO 2005

INTERNATIONAL STANDARD
ISO/IEC 17025

Second edition 2005-05-15

General requirements for the competence of testing and calibration laboratories

Exigences générales concernant la compétence des laboratoires d'étalonnages et d'essais

Foreword

ISO (the International Organization for Standardization) and IEC (the International Electrotechnical Commission) form the specialized system for worldwide standardization. National bodies that are members of ISO or IEC participate in the development of International Standards through technical committees established by the respective organization to deal with particular fields of technical activity. ISO and IEC technical committees collaborate in fields of mutual interest. Other international organizations, governmental and non-governmental, in liaison with ISO and IEC, also take part in the work. In the field of conformity assessment, the ISO Committee on conformity assessment (CASCO) is responsible for the development of International Standards and Guides.

International Standards are drafted in accordance with the rules given in the ISO/IEC Directives, Part 2.

Draft International Standards are circulated to the national bodies for voting. Publication as an International Standard requires approval by at least 75% of the national bodies casting a vote.

Attention is drawn to the possibility that some of the elements of this document may be the subject of patent rights. ISO shall not be held responsible for identifying any or all such patent rights.

ISO/IEC 17025 was prepared by the *ISO Committee on conformity assessment* (CASCO).

It was circulated for voting to the national bodies of both ISO and IEC, and was approved by both organizations.

This second edition cancels and replaces the first edition (ISO/IEC 17025:1999), which has been technically revised.

Introduction

The first edition (1999) of this International Standard was produced as the result of extensive experience in the implementation of ISO/IEC Guide 25 and EN 45001, both of which it replaced. It contained all of the requirements that testing and calibration laboratories have to meet if they wish to demonstrate that they operate a management system, are technically competent, and are able to generate technically valid results.

The first edition referred to ISO 9001:1994 and ISO 9002:1994. These standards have been superseded by ISO 9001:2000, which made an alignment of ISO/IEC 17025 necessary. In this second edition, clauses have been amended or added only when considered necessary in the light of ISO 9001:2000.

Accreditation bodies that recognize the competence of testing and calibration laboratories should use this International Standard as the basis for their accreditation. Clause 4 specifies the requirements for sound management. Clause 5 specifies the requirements for technical competence for the type of tests and/or calibrations the laboratory undertakes.

Growth in the use of management systems generally has increased the need to ensure that laboratories which form part of larger organizations or offer other services can operate to a quality management system that is seen as compliant with ISO 9001 as well as with this International Standard. Care has been taken, therefore, to incorporate all those requirements of ISO 9001 that are relevant to the scope of testing and calibration services that are covered by the laboratory's management system.

Testing and calibration laboratories that comply with this International Standard will therefore also operate in accordance with ISO 9001.

Conformity of the quality management system within which the laboratory operates to the requirements of ISO 9001 does not of itself demonstrate the competence of the laboratory to produce technically valid data and results. Nor does demonstrated conformity to this International Standard imply conformity of the quality management system within which the laboratory operates to all the requirements of ISO 9001.

The acceptance of testing and calibration results between countries should be facilitated if laboratories comply with this International Standard and if they obtain accreditation from bodies which have entered into mutual recognition agreements with equivalent bodies in other countries using this International Standard.

The use of this International Standard will facilitate cooperation between laboratories and other bodies, and assist in the exchange of information and experience, and in the harmonization of standards and procedures.

General requirements for the competence of testing and calibration laboratories

1 Scope

1.1 This International Standard specifies the general requirements for the competence to carry out tests and/or calibrations, including sampling. It covers testing and calibration performed using standard methods, non-standard methods, and laboratory-developed methods.

1.2 This International Standard is applicable to all organizations performing tests and/or calibrations. These include, for example, first-, second- and third-party laboratories, and laboratories where testing and/or calibration forms part of inspection and product certification.

This International Standard is applicable to all laboratories regardless of the number of personnel or the extent of the scope of testing and/or calibration activities. When a laboratory does not undertake one or more of the activities covered by this International Standard, such as sampling and the design/development of new methods, the requirements of those clauses do not apply.

1.3 The notes given provide clarification of the text, examples and guidance. They do not contain requirements and do not form an integral part of this International Standard.

1.4 This International Standard is for use by laboratories in developing their management system for quality, administrative and technical operations. Laboratory customers, regulatory authorities and accreditation bodies may also use it in confirming or recognizing the competence of laboratories. This International Standard is not intended to be used as the basis for certification of laboratories.

NOTE 1 The term 'management system' in this International Standard means the quality, administrative and technical systems that govern the operations of a laboratory.

NOTE 2 Certification of a management system is sometimes also called registration.

1.5 Compliance with regulatory and safety requirements on the operation of laboratories is not covered by this International Standard.

1.6 If testing and calibration laboratories comply with the requirements of this International Standard, they will operate a quality management system for their testing and calibration activities that also meets the principles of ISO 9001. Annex A provides nominal cross-references between this International Standard and ISO 9001. This International Standard covers technical competence requirements that are not covered by ISO 9001.

NOTE 1 It might be necessary to explain or interpret certain requirements in this International Standard to ensure that the requirements are applied in a consistent manner. Guidance for establishing applications for specific fields, especially for accreditation bodies (see ISO/IEC 17011) is given in Annex B.

NOTE 2 If a laboratory wishes accreditation for part or all of its testing and calibration activities, it should select an accreditation body that operates in accordance with ISO/IEC 17011.

Authors' Forensic Management Research

The transition from craft-based, labor-intensive work to more automated systems has impacted employee recruitment, selection, and training in the forensic sciences. In this technologically fluid environment the trend is toward increased specialization, with routine collection of evidence shifting to police personnel in the field. *CSI* aside, forensic science jobs lack the glamour portrayed in the media. The difficulty attracting and retaining competent forensic scientists in public crime labs within the constraints of the civil service system was noted a half century ago. Salaries not competitive with the private sector are associated with chronic staff shortages and employee turnover.

We find crime labs interesting and unusual organizations to study. The work environment consists of a zero tolerance for mistakes, an unpredictable work flow, and constant backlogs. Labs are hierarchical, quasi-military operations, typically housed within police departments. Agency demands can divert attention from the needs of the lab in favor of patrol vehicles and police officers. Forensic scientists often report to sworn officers, who may not fully understand the technical scientific issues. There are often no career paths provided for forensic scientists, other than the police ranks of lieutenant, captain, major.

Team structures offer advantages yet remain underutilized. As an example, DNA processing currently involves an inefficient boutique method of casework analysis: one scientist performs all tasks needed to complete the case. In contrast, the implementation of high performance team models along with recent innovations in batch processing and computer expert systems would dramatically improve productivity. A multidiscipline case might involve ballistic, hair, fiber, and DNA evidence analyses; a project team would ensure collaboration between technical disciplines and facilitate communication with management.

Increased lab productivity helps stop criminals earlier in their criminal careers. The implicit theory is that offenders identified as a result of minor criminal activity do not advance to more serious crime because many convicted offenders have previously committed minor crimes. The implication for well-staffed, quality-driven crime labs includes a reduction of crime nationwide. The articles summarized below are representative of our research involving employee management issues in the forensic sciences. To read the full text of these articles, please visit *www.fbi.gov/hq/lab/fsc/current/backissu.htm.*

"Critical Human Resource Issues: Scientists Under Pressure" presents a national survey of forensic science laboratory managers. Issues such as the importance of level of staffing, outsourcing, and the pressures experienced by forensic scientists, are examined in detail. We expect that the answers to these challenges will become increasingly important as incentives to outsource forensic activities from the public to the private sector increases.

"Managing Intellectual Capital" describes the strategy of providing a forensic advisory group for on-the-job professional development. Forensic advisory groups consist of experienced and retired forensic professionals from various technical disciplines and the academic community; members are chosen for their ability to build trust and share knowledge with laboratory staff. Available through phone calls, e-mails and review meetings, forensic advisory group members help to create a culture of mentoring and collaboration for staff, who may otherwise be isolated. The forensic advisory group resides in the lab for a specified period of time (for example, one week), providing developmental feedback to employees. Coaching is provided for testifying scientists to build their confidence in court. Further analysis is needed of the relationship between innovative management strategies, such as forensic advisory groups, and lab outcomes.

"A Case Study of Forensic Scientist Turnover" examines employee issues in a large northeastern state crime lab. Typically, intense on-the-job apprenticeships of at least one year are required to develop forensic scientists. During this time, senior scientists can experience productivity declines of up to 50 percent while they train new employees. A staffing model was created with a new support position of laboratory technician that would perform routine duties in the lab, so that data interpretation and more complex tasks could be reserved for scientists. The two-tiered structure proposed saving the organization $1 million. After one year, 16 of 53 newly hired employees left the organization. Costs associated with the early departure of these employees exceeded the estimated savings, and the experiment was considered a failure. Exit interviews revealed that laboratory technicians had anticipated a rapid move into forensic scientist positions. However, when they learned that promotional opportunities were limited, employees quickly left the organization, often for private sector jobs.

"Strategic Human Resource Management in the Forensic Science Laboratory" provides staffing strategies for managers of crime labs. Realistic job previews can be used more extensively in this industry, to supplement extensive use of pre-employment testing. Professional development opportunities are also recommended for retaining technical workers. This can include tuition reimbursement, flexible work hours, and attendance at professional meetings, seminars, and conferences. In addition, training in more than one discipline, such as a primary area like latent prints, and a secondary area, like footprints, can be used as an incentive for employees.

The 21st century is the century of DNA, bringing profound change. The future will see expansion of internationally integrated databases with accelerated testing and increased miniaturization of evidence samples. Tele-forensics, data mining, digital documentation, and expert system models are already on the horizon. Management factors are important to complement the impressive advances in crime lab technology. The future of this industry depends on overcoming case backlogs and increased demand for services, transitioning to automated systems, and making the best use of information databases and new technology. Well-educated, trained, and competent employees are critical to this vision.

References

Becker, W. S., and W. M. Dale. 2007. Critical human resource issues: Scientists under pressure. *Forensic Science Communications* 9 (2). *www.fbi.gov/hq/lab/fsc/backissu/april2007/research/2007_04_research02.htm*

Becker, W. S., and W. M. Dale. 2003. Strategic human resource management in the forensic science laboratory. *Forensic Science Communications* 5 (4). *www.fbi.gov/hq/lab/fsc/backissu/oct2003/2003_10_research01.htm*

Dale, W. M., and W. S. Becker. 2005. Managing intellectual capital. *Forensic Science Communications* 7 (4). *www.fbi.gov/hq/lab/fsc/ backissu/oct2005/research/2005_10_research02.htm*

Dale, W. M., and W. S. Becker. 2004. A case study of forensic scientist turnover. *Forensic Science Communications* 6 (4). *www.fbi.gov/hq/ lab/fsc/backissu/july2004/research/2004_03_research04.htm*

PHOTO CREDITS

"Edmond Locard" Courtesy of Microtrace LLC "Lab technicians preparing DNA extracts" Courtesy of W. Mark Dale "Two bullets viewed from a comparison microscope" Courtesy of State of Connecticut Department of Public Safety "Automated Fingerprint Identification System" Courtesy of Ed German, onin.com/ed "Scientist using microscope to recognize evidence" Courtesy of W. Mark Dale "An emergency response team at the scene" Courtesy of Sandia National Laboratories "Fingerprint Powders" Courtesy of BUDA International "First responders" Courtesy of Sandia National Laboratories "Crime scene team" Courtesy of W. Mark Dale "Evidence recovery team" Courtesy of the FBI Laboratory of Quantico, VA "Portable swipe analysis tool" Courtesy of Sandia National Laboratories "Fingerprint processed with superglue" Courtesy of Greg Grieco "Decontaminating biological agents" Courtesy of Sandia National Laboratories "Evidence is collected, labeled, and photographed before going to the lab" Courtesy of Richard T. Davis, Danville Register and Bee "Evidence collection kit" Courtesy of Don O'Neil, Sirchie Labs, Inc. "Handheld device/portable lab" Courtesy of Sandia National Laboratories "Dusting for latent prints" Courtesy of Hans van den Nieuwendijk "The fingerprints of Francisco Rojas, the first person convicted of murder through fingerprint evidence" Courtesy of The National Library of Medicine at the the National Institutes of Health "Latent print from non-porous surface" Courtesy of BVDA International BV "Forensic scientist cutting swab from blood soaked garment" Courtesy of W. Mark Dale "Scientist pipetting biological fluids" Courtesy of the FBI Laboratory of Quantico, VA "Forged check" Courtesy of San Diego County Sheriff's Department Crime Lab "Confocal microscopy" Courtesy of W. Mark Dale "Research on fibers" Courtesy of W. Mark Dale "Analysis of projectile in motion" Courtesy of State of Connecticut Department of Public Safety "Firearm muzzle blast" Courtesy of Andrew Davidhazy, Rochester Institute of Technology "Microscopic view of damaged hair" "Microscopic view of raised cuticle hair" "Microscopic view of healthy hair" "Cross-sectional microscopic view of hair" and "Showing a different texture of hair" all Courtesy of the FBI Laboratory of Quantico, VA "Milt Helpern, former chief medical examiner, New York City" Courtesy of The National Library of Medicine at the the National Institutes of Health "Forensic pathologist" Courtesy of Thomas Wright from the University of Florida/IFAS "Autopsy tools" Courtesy of BVDA International BV "Human skull with foreign objects: How did those get there?" Courtesy of Vidisco Ltd. the Portable X-ray manufacturer "Medical examiner body diagrams" Courtesy of Armed Forces Institute of Pathology "Ohio death certificate" Courtesy of Jackie Higgins Chan "Body diagram with notes" Courtesy of Jackie Higgins Chan "Autopsy notes" Courtesy of Jackie Higgins Chan "Autopsy suite" Courtesy of the FBI Laboratory of Quantico, VA "Bar codes are used for inventory and chain of custody" Courtesy of Sandia National Laboratories "Bar code provides unique case identifier" Courtesy of Sandia National Laboratories "Drug detection electron microscope" Courtesy of Sandia National Laboratories "DNA scientist" Courtesy of the FBI Laboratory of Quantico, VA "Microscopic visualization of evidence" Courtesy of W. Mark Dale "Pipetting DNA extractions" Courtesy of the FBI Laboratory of Quantico, VA "DNA analysis instrumentation" Courtesy of W. Mark Dale "DNA data interpretation" Courtesy of W. Mark Dale "DNA technical leader reviewing casework data" Courtesy of W. Mark Dale "DNA was used to identify victims of the WTC disaster" Courtesy of Shawn Moore/OSHA News "Sanitized laboratory tools" Courtesy of W. Mark Dale "Scientist operating centrifuge" Courtesy of W. Mark Dale "Scientist pipetting DNA extracts" Courtesy of W. Mark Dale "Firearms are test-fired into water tanks" Courtesy of California Association of Criminalists "Lands and grooves within barrel of gun" Courtesy of Georgia Bureau of Investigation, Department of Forensic Sciences "Land and groove impressions on projectile" Courtesy of Georgia Bureau of Investigation, Department of Forensic Sciences "Ballistic comparisons" Courtesy of The Public Information and Education Division of the Missouri State Highway Patrol "Fiber" Courtesy of Laboratory of John Badding, Penn State University "Matching fibers in duct tape" Courtesy of the FBI Laboratory of Quantico, VA "Fiber research" Courtesy of W. Mark Dale "Case triage team" Courtesy of Richard T. Davis, Danville Register and Bee "Prosecutor in court" Courtesy of Northeast Regional Forensics Institute (NERFI) "Typical courtroom" Courtesy of the Bernard Weitzman Model Courtroom at William Woods University "Courtroom" Courtesy of the Bernard Weitzman Model Courtroom at William Woods University "New technology" Courtesy of Sandia National Laboratories "DNA helix" Courtesy of Wayne Heim "Computer crime" Courtesy of Sandia National Laboratories "First responder with PDA and Haz-mat gear" Courtesy of Sandia National Laboratories "Training" Courtesy of Sandia National Laboratories "Gunshot residue collection" Courtesy of Sandia National Laboratories "Fluorescing Fingerprints" Courtesy of Sandia National Laboratories "Fiber research with laser" Courtesy of W. Mark Dale "Crime scene team" Courtesy of Richard T. Davis, Danville Register and Bee "Mobile and stationary evidence storage systems" Courtesy of W. Mark Dale

INDEX

A

AAFS. *See* American Academy of Forensic Sciences
Abandonment, 118
ABC. *See* American Board of Criminalistics
Accidental death, 88
Acetaminophen, 139
Adhesive, 58
Adhesive tape, 56
Adjacent areas, 36
AFIS. *See* Automated Fingerprint Identification System
AFTE. *See* Association of Firearm and Tool Mark Examiners
Alcohol, 97, 101
Alcohol, Tobacco, Firearms and Explosives, Bureau of (ATF), 3, 129, 134, 176
Algor mortis, 89
Aluminum powder, 64
American Academy of Forensic Sciences (AAFS), 199, 200, 201
American Board of Criminalistics (ABC), 202
American Society of Crime Laboratory Directors/ Laboratory Accreditation Board (ASCLD/LAB), 31,

134, 183, 188–89, 199, 200, 201
Amido black, 58, 64
Ammunition, 71–74
Amphetamines, 139
Analogies, 167
Animal hair, 143
Anthropologist, 26
Approach, crime scene, 34
Ardrox, 58
Aronson, H., 85
Arsenic, 82, 97
Artificial heart valve, 96
Asbestos, 97
ASCLD/LAB. *See* American Society of Crime Laboratory Directors/Laboratory Accreditation Board
Assignments, 32–33
Association of Firearm and Tool Mark Examiners (AFTE), 130
ATF. *See* Alcohol, Tobacco, Firearms and Explosives, Bureau of
Attendance log, 17, 19, 34
Audio solutions, 185
Autolysis, 91
Automated Fingerprint Identification System (AFIS), xiii, xiv, 3, 5, 162, 175, 185
Automobile searches, 165
Autopsy, x, 81

coroner vs. medical examiner, 86–87
dissection, 91–96
documentation maintenance, 97
evidence, 85–86
information assessed at, 88–91
notes, 94

B

Bacon, Francis, 152–53
Bacterial degradation, 35
Bag and tag, 25, 73
Bailey, F. Lee, 85
Ballistic
analyses, 157
comparisons, 132–33, 134, 135
wounds, 61
Barbiturates, 139
Bar codes, 107, 108, 109
Batch processing, xi
Becker, Wendy, xiii
Benzodiazepines, 139
Big picture, 7, 31
Biohazard containers, 60
Biohazards, 47
Biological evidence, 109
detection, 50
materials, 62

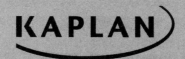
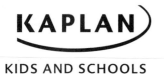
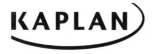
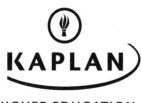
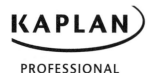